Questions & A̶ Sleep A̶

Sudhansu Chokroverty, MD, FRCP, FACP

Professor and Co-Chair of Neurology
Program Director,
Clinical Neurophysiology & Sleep Medicine .
New Jersey Neuroscience Institute at JFK
Seton Hall University
Edison, NJ

JONES AND BARTLETT PUBLISHERS
Sudbury, Massachusetts
BOSTON   TORONTO   LONDON   SINGAPORE

World Headquarters

Jones and Bartlett Publishers
40 Tall Pine Drive
Sudbury, MA 01776
978-443-5000
info@jbpub.com
www.jbpub.com

Jones and Bartlett Publishers
Canada
6339 Ormindale Way
Mississauga, Ontario L5V 1J2
Canada

Jones and Bartlett Publishers
International
Barb House, Barb Mews
London W6 7PA
United Kingdom

Jones and Bartlett's books and products are available through most bookstores and online book-sellers. To contact Jones and Bartlett Publishers directly, call 800-832-0034, fax 978-443-8000, or visit our website, www.jbpub.com.

Substantial discounts on bulk quantities of Jones and Bartlett's publications are available to cor-porations, professional associations, and other qualified organizations. For details and specific discount information, contact the special sales department at Jones and Bartlett via the above contact information or send an email to specialsales@jbpub.com.

The authors, editor, and publisher have made every effort to provide accurate information. However, they are not responsible for errors, omissions, or for any outcomes related to the use of the contents of this book and take no responsibility for the use of the products and procedures described. Treat-ments and side effects described in this book may not be applicable to all people; likewise, some peo-ple may require a dose or experience a side effect that is not described herein. Drugs and medical devices are discussed that may have limited availability controlled by the Food and Drug Adminis-tration (FDA) for use only in a research study or clinical trial. Research, clinical practice, and gov-ernment regulations often change the accepted standard in this field. When consideration is being given to use of any drug in the clinical setting, the health care provider or reader is responsible for determining FDA status of the drug, reading the package insert, and reviewing prescribing informa-tion for the most up-to-date recommendations on dose, precautions, and contraindications, and determining the appropriate usage for the product. This is especially important in the case of drugs that are new or seldom used.

Production Credits
Executive Publisher: Christopher Davis
Custom Projects Editor: Kathy Richardson
Sr. Editorial Assistant: Jessica Acox
Associate Production Editor: Leah Corrigan
Associate Marketing Manager: Ilana Goddess
Manufacturing and Inventory Control Supervisor: Amy Bacus
Composition: Northeast Compositors, Inc.
Cover Design: Kristin E. Ohlin
Cover Image: © Steve Luker/Shutterstock, Inc.
    Courtesy of ResMed
Printing and Binding: Malloy, Inc.
Cover Printing: Malloy, Inc.

Library of Congress Cataloging-in-Publication Data
Chokroverty, Sudhansu.
    Questions and answers about sleep apnea / Sudhansu Chokroverty.
        p. cm.
    ISBN 978-0-7637-6377-0
    1. Sleep apnea syndromes--Popular works. I. Title.
    RC737.5.C56 2009
    616.2'09--dc22

6048   2008019410

Printed in the United States of America
12 11 10 09 08   10 9 8 7 6 5 4 3 2 1

Contents

1. What is sleep?
2. What is the purpose of sleep?
3. How much sleep do I need?
4. How common are sleep problems?
5. I was told by my wife that I snore a lot. Why do I snore? Does snoring mean that I have sleep apnea? Or is it just a nuisance?
6. My wife tells me I snore loudly, driving her crazy. I also feel sleepy in the daytime. Should I use a snore guard or see a doctor?
7. How does sleep affect breathing in a normal person?
8. Is snoring related to any physical defect? Can snoring cause any physical illness or memory impairment?
9. I am a 65-year-old man falling asleep in the daytime in inappropriate places and under inappropriate circumstances. I have been in one minor car accident and have almost been in two other car accidents because of the excessive sleepiness. Should I see my primary physician or a sleep specialist?

10. What is sleep apnea?
11. What are the clues that I should look for if I think I have sleep apnea?
12. Can sleep apnea run in the family?
13. How are the normal breathing events during sleep changed in sleep apnea?
14. Why is snoring or sleep apnea worse after drinking alcohol or taking a sleeping medication?
15. My friend told me that sleep apnea is a serious condition that may cause both short- and long-term serious consequences. Is my friend correct?
16. I have heard that people with sleep apnea may die suddenly in the middle of the night. Is this true?
17. My doctor recently noted that I have high blood pressure. She began treatment but is having difficulty controlling the blood pressure level. I also snore. Can this problem with my blood pressure be due to sleep apnea?

Part 3: Diagnosing Sleep Apnea   37

Part 4: Treating Sleep Apnea   55

Part 5: Living with Sleep Apnea   85

There is now increasing evidence that sleep apnea (transient cessation of breathing during sleep) may cause high blood pressure, coronary arterial disease, stroke, and memory impairment. Sleep apnea may be considered a silent epidemic that often remains undiagnosed or under-diagnosed. There is, however, reluctance to accept these grim facts. People are not taking sleep disorders, including sleep apnea, seriously. This is not just a United States attitude, but also a global phenomenon. This must be rectified by educating the public as well as physicians not specializing in sleep medicine, because there is now effective treatment available to avert the disastrous consequences of sleep apnea, sleep deprivation, and other sleep dysfunctions.

It is interesting to note that this condition (sleep apnea) was brought to our attention, not by a physician, but by a famous English writer, Charles Dickens, in the 19th century. In the posthumous papers of the Pickwick Club the author described Joe as "the fat boy" who is always sleepy and snoring while falling asleep. This is reminiscent of the modern description of a patient with sleep apnea, which is associated with obesity in about 70% of cases. The medical community waited until the middle of the 20th century when Auchincloss, Burwell, and co-investigators (1955-56) from the United States dubbed the condition *Pickwickian syndrome*. It was, however, two groups of neurologists from France (Gastaut and Tassinari) and Germany (Kuhlo and Jung) who independently identified the site of the obstruction responsible for sleep apnea in the upper airway. This was quickly followed by effective treatment of sleep apnea, first by tracheostomy (making a hole in front of the neck to bypass the site of obstruction to airflow in the upper airway) and next by the discovery of continuous positive airway pressure (CPAP) in 1981 by Sullivan from Australia. The rest is history. We now have an effective treatment for this potentially serious disorder, and as physicians it is our responsibility to educate the public and the profession so that we can help a large segment of the population (about 15–20 million individuals in the United States alone) suffering from sleep apnea. I hope this little booklet discussing the condition in a question and answer format contributes toward these goals in a small way.

Sudhansu Chokroverty, MD, FRCP, FACP

Acknowledgments

It is my pleasure to acknowledge some of the individuals who helped bring this book out. First and foremost, I thank my wife, Manisha Chokroverty, MD, for her forbearance, patience, and for contributing some of the questions in this monograph.

I must thank Betty Coram for typing and Annabella Drennan for editing and making corrections. Finally, I am indebted to Christopher Davis, Executive Publisher, Medicine; Kathy Richardson, Associate Editor; and Edward Staples, Marketing Manager at Jones and Bartlett Publishers for their professionalism and dedication, without whom this book would not have seen the light of day.

Sudhansu Chokroverty, MD, FRCP, FACP

I never appreciated the importance of getting enough good sleep until I started working in the sleep apnea field.

I had heard of sleep apnea before and, like most people, I thought it was a condition that affected middle-aged, overweight men. I thought, again like most people, it came from making poor lifestyle choices—too much junk food and too much time sitting on the couch watching television. Boy, was I mistaken!

Sleep and breathing are two bodily functions that we take for granted. Try as we might to avoid sleeping, eventually it catches up with us—though, hopefully not while behind the wheel of a moving automobile.

If you don't breathe—you die. It's that simple. The brain goes to great lengths to keep the gas exchange in the lungs going—oxygen for carbon dioxide in the blood.

Now bring these two processes together, imagine falling asleep, your body relaxes as it moves into the deeper, more restorative stages of sleep. All the muscles and tissues relax, including those that surround the only opening where air enters the lungs, causing an obstruction. The blockage results in no air entering the lungs and no oxygen entering the blood. This continues until the build-up of CO_2 in the bloodstream is intolerable and the brain rouses the body to start breathing again. You then return to a lighter stage of sleep.

Imagine if this happens 30, 40, 50, or more times per hour. This is sleep apnea.

The combination of sleep fragmentation and recurring spikes in blood pressure results in a proverbial Pandora's box of bad health consequences. These problems can be cardiovascular (high blood pressure leading to heart disease), metabolic (exacerbating diabetes), and psychological (depression, reduced quality of life).

In my experience as the Executive Director of the American Sleep Apnea Association I have seen the effects of untreated sleep apnea reaching beyond the individual, similar to the expanding circle after dropping a pebble into a pond. Living with untreated sleep apnea significantly affects the life of the sufferer—both quality and quantity.

But it does not stop there. Anyone sleeping with the sufferer has his or her own sleep interrupted. Other members of the family may be subjected to increased irritability of the person with the condition.

The circle of misery expands further to include the workplace. The untreated apneic is frequently less productive because of excessive daytime sleepiness. The sufferer can be more costly to their employer as a result of accidents and higher healthcare utilization.

Finally, at its widest point the circle engulfs the larger society when industrial accidents due to inattention from lack of sleep occur. These have an impact that extends far beyond the confines of the workplace.

Sleep apnea affects a significant percentage of the adult population. Serious as it is, it is easily diagnosed and treated.

In what follows, Dr. Chokroverty provides answers to 60 of the more important questions about this disease. Reading this book is an important first step in treating your sleep apnea or that of a loved one.

Edward Grandi
Executive Director
American Sleep Apnea Association
Washington, DC

Hi, I'm Andy, and I snore. I snore so badly that ten years ago an entire hunting camp full of 60-year-old men told me that I was the world champion snorer of all time. For a long time, I laughed and dismissed their comments.

Then I got married. My wife told me I snore, too. I snore so badly that my wife had to wear earplugs to bed. Even with the earplugs, I'd get an elbow in the ribs, or she'd give me a shake to get me to roll over so I wasn't snoring in her direction. Some mornings, I'd get dirty looks over coffee (which I *really* needed) because I'd kept her up with my snoring.

Then we had kids. Believe it or not, kids make you tired. New parents keep hours that would make college students tired; 2:00 a.m. feedings, 4:00 a.m. feedings. Your entire sleep rhythm gets thrown off. Now I'm a night owl by nature, and I know I don't always get *enough* sleep. What I didn't know was that the sleep I was getting wasn't letting me get the rest I really needed.

Sleep apnea snuck up on me. One day last year, my daughter asked me why I kept hitting the rumble strips on the edge of the highway. I was a drowsy driver, and every time I got behind the wheel, I was putting myself, my family, and everyone else at risk. If I hadn't done something about my sleep apnea, I might have killed someone by falling asleep at the wheel.

After reading some information, and talking with my doctor, I went to have a sleep study. Within the first two hours of falling asleep, they were certain that I had sleep apnea. Sixty events an hour. It was pretty serious.

My sleep technician provided me with a CPAP machine, and it has made all the difference. The silicone mask is very comfortable. It "floats" on your face on the air cushion from the machine. The straps are just tight enough to keep it from shifting around. It took me about a week to get used to sleeping while wearing the mask, and now I can't imagine sleeping without it. I don't even notice that I'm wearing it anymore.

With my CPAP, I no longer snore. Now I get the rest I need, my blood pressure has dropped ten points on both scores, my wife can sleep without earplugs again, and I no longer *need* those first two cups of coffee to get going in the morning.

I still need to get *more* sleep, but with my CPAP, I'm getting the quality rest that I need to function and be healthy.

PART ONE

Sleep Basics

What is sleep?

How much sleep should I have?

How does sleep affect breathing in a normal person?

More ...

1. What is sleep?

The phenomenon of sleep includes both passive mechanisms—for example, withdrawal of all external and internal stimulation—and active mechanisms. Sleep is not simply an absence of wakefulness and perception, nor is it just a passive phenomenon resulting from withdrawal of all sensory stimuli. Many areas of the brain remain active during sleep. All the structures responsible for generating sleep and wakefulness are located within the brain. Sleep contributes to your overall health, affecting not only the brain but also the entire body, as evidenced by the many diseases that may result from too much sleep, too little sleep, inappropriate timing of sleep, or abnormal movements and behaviors intruding into sleep. There are many chemicals sending signals to different groups of nerve cells in the brain switching off or switching on certain groups of neurons determining the sleep and wakefulness.

Many areas of the brain remain active during sleep.

The word "sleep" is derived from the Latin word *somnus*, the German word *slaf*, and the Greek word *hypnos*. Although sleep has aroused the interest of mankind since time immemorial, as reflected in the writings of the eastern and western religions and civilizations, the mystical nature of sleep and the definition of sleep have eluded the philosophers, religious scholars, scientists, and poets throughout the ages. Most realistically, this question of what sleep is should be asked when one is trying to get to sleep. But it is difficult to ask this question when we lie down, close our eyes, and try to forget about the world of wakefulness. Slowly we begin drifting to a state beyond wakefulness when we do not see, hear, or perceive things in a rational or logical manner. We are now in another world, where we have no control, our brain cannot respond logically and adequately, and our body is relatively immobile. We are now entering what is termed **predormitum**. Soon we are drifting from lighter to deeper stages of sleep. We are now unconscious. Fortunately, this state is reversible—a characteristic that differentiates sleep from irreversible coma (complete unconsciousness as a result of a disease) and death. Sleep in fact is referred as the brother of death in the classic literature (Homer's *Iliad*, circa 700 B.C.). We will wake up to see the world of wakefulness after about seven or eight hours of sleep. Most of us go to sleep at night (unless we work a night shift). We finish our day's activities, and after relaxing in the evening, we prepare to go to sleep. It is interesting to note, as Roger Ekirch wrote in his fascinating book *At Day's Close*, that centuries before the discovery of light and electricity, night sleep habits of mankind were different from the consolidated sleep we seek nowadays. In the days past, there were two periods of sleep at night consisting of four hours at a stretch with a break of two to three hours in between. This interval was occupied with planning, dreaming, intimacy, meditating, and visiting.

Humans, animals, and plants all follow a basic rest-activity pattern that occurs in cycles synchronized with fluctuations of darkness and sunlight and is a fundamental rhythmicity in all living organisms. The rotation of the Earth determines the timing of both the rest-activity cycle and the sleep-wakefulness rhythm.

Predormitum

A state of diminished perception and control through which a person passes in progressing from wakefulness into the sleep state.

Sleep Basics

Sleep-wake habits are controlled not only by external light and darkness as determined by sunrise and sunset but also by our internal body clock. This question of an internal body clock was first raised more than two and a half centuries ago by a French astronomer named de Mairin. He noticed that the leaves of a heliotrope plant would open at sunrise and close at sunset, even when the plant was kept inside away from sunlight. This observation led de Mairin to conclude that an internal clock in the plant must control the opening and closing of the leaves. Only toward the end of the twentieth century did scientists discover the existence of an internal clock in rats and shortly thereafter confirm that such a clock operates in humans as well. This human internal clock is thought to reside within a cluster of nerve cells (called **suprachiasmatic nuclei**) located deep in the center of the brain above the **pituitary gland**, the organ that is responsible for secretion of several important hormones. This internal clock has widespread connections, not only with the **retina** (nerve cell layer in the back of the eye) for receiving light from the outside world but also with other parts of the nervous system. As a result, it controls the body's sleep-wake cycle, secretion of hormones, and the temperature rhythms.

The modern definition of sleep is based on the behavior of the person while asleep and the physiological changes that occur in the waking brain as one is drifting into sleep. The behavioral criteria include a characteristic posture, relative immobility, reduced response to external stimulation, and closed eyes. The physiological criteria define the various sleep stages and

Suprachiasmatic nuclei

A cluster of nerve cells within which the human internal clock is thought to reside.

Pituitary gland

The organ responsible for secretion of several important hormones.

Retina

The layer of nerve cells at the back of the eye responsible for transmitting visual images to the back of the brain.

states and are based on recording of electrical activities of the brain (through an **electroencephalogram**, or **EEG**), the muscles (through an **electromyogram**, or **EMG**), and eye movements (through an **electrooculogram**, or **EOG**).

Sleep is broadly divided into two states: **non-rapid eye movement (NREM) sleep** and **rapid eye movement (REM) sleep**. NREM sleep is traditionally subdivided into four stages that have been slightly modified in a recent revision combining traditional stages 3 and 4 into stage N3 only. In stage 1, the predominant wakeful brain rhythm of an adult decreases to less than half of that seen in the wakeful state. The muscle tone decreases a little and some rolling, slow eye movements take place. In stage 2 NREM sleep, brain electrical activity shows a characteristic pattern called **sleep spindles** (brain rhythms of 11 to 16, most commonly 14, cycles per second that are seen in surface recordings taken from the front and center of the head). The sleep spindles are accompanied by slower waves (less than four cycles per second) during less than 20% of the time. The slow wave or deep sleep, which is a combination of traditional stages 3 and 4 or the recent revision called stage N3, is dominated by brain waves slower than four cycles per second. Most of our time during sleep is spent in stage 2 NREM sleep. There is an orderly progression of sleep pattern in a normal adult human being. Approximately five to ten minutes after sleep onset, we drift from stage 1 to stage 2, and then after about one hour, we go into slow wave sleep. About 60 to 90 minutes after sleep onset, we enter into the world of dream sleep—that is, REM sleep, the

Electroencephalogram (EEG)

A recording of the electrical activities of the brain.

Electromyogram (EMG)

A recording of the electrical activities of the muscles.

Electro-oculogram (EOG)

A recording of the movements of the eye.

Non-rapid eye movement (NREM) sleep

The multi-stage phase of the progression from wakefulness into deep sleep.

Rapid eye movement (REM) sleep

The stage of sleep during which dreaming occurs.

Sleep spindles

Brain rhythms of 14 to 16 cycles per second that are seen in surface recordings taken from the front and center of the head during NREM sleep.

Sleep Basics

state in which most dreams occur. Eyeballs may move rapidly under the closed eyelids; hence the name "rapid eye movement" sleep. Muscle tone in the EMG recording decreases markedly or is absent, and the brain waves (shown on the EEG) resemble those noted during wakefulness. NREM and REM sleep alternate in a cyclical manner (about four to six cycles) interspersed with brief periods of wakefulness throughout the night. During the first third of the night, slow-wave sleep dominates; conversely, during the last third of the night, REM sleep dominates. REM sleep accounts for 20% to 25% of the sleep period in human adults. Different sleep patterns, including the time occupied by different stages of sleep, are observed in newborns, children, and the elderly.

2. What is the purpose of sleep?

The function of sleep has been debated throughout the centuries without an adequate answer. Recent evidence shows that both the brain and the rest of the body need an optimal amount of sleep. If we do not have adequate sleep at night, we feel sleepy, irritable, and awful throughout the day. Although the exact function of sleep is not known, we know that sleep is necessary for survival. Several theories have been proposed based on the results of animal and human **sleep deprivation** experiments. For example, we may require sleep for energy conservation and for restoration of the body and brain that allows them to function adequately during the waking period. It has been suggested that sleep is needed for both consolidation and reconsolidation of memory (restoration of lost memory after the period

Sleep deprivation

The condition of sleeplessness resulting in sleep debt and other adverse consequences.

of sleep) and for adequate stimulation of various nerve circuits within the brain that ensure proper functioning. Human experiments have shown that recent facts that have been forgotten during acute sleep deprivation can be restored after a period of sleep. Recent evidence also suggests that different genes (expression of proteins) are transcripted in the brain during sleep and wakefulness, indicating different functions of the brain during these two states. We also know that deep sleep promotes the release of growth hormone, which is very important for children and young adults. In addition, production of new proteins in the brain during sleep may promote cell growth. Sleep may also provide for regulation of body temperature. Although we do not know its exact function, sleep is critical for survival and for maintaining good physical and mental health.

3. How much sleep do I need?

The basic human sleep requirement depends on your age and is defined by heredity rather than by any environmental influence. The average requirement for a normal adult man or woman is approximately seven and a half to eight hours. Sleep requirements, just like many behavioral functions and requirements, assume a bell-shaped curve. Thus, some people require less than the average amount of sleep and some require more sleep to function adequately during waking hours. Some individuals can get by with six to seven hours of sleep (or less), whereas others require nine to ten hours of sleep each night. Newborns need 16 hours of sleep a day. This requirement decreases to about ten hours by about three to five years of age. Old age is marked by repeated awakenings throughout the night and napping during the daytime, but the total duration of sleep time during a 24-hour period is no different from that of a middle-aged adult. A common misperception is that everyone must have seven and a half to eight hours of sleep, otherwise they will not be able to function during the daytime. The ideal sleep requirement is the amount of sleep you need to feel rested, refreshed, and energetic on awakening in the morning and ready to function adequately.

4. How common are sleep problems?

Sleep problems are very common, as epidemiological surveys undertaken in the United States and other parts of the world as well as day-to-day practice in sleep medicine have made it abundantly clear. A report by the National Commission of Sleep Disorders Research in 1993 stated that millions of Americans are affected by sleep disorders, costing society billions of dollars. This report galvanized the sleep community, the public, and branches of medical professions, and there is now a growing perception of sleep problems among the public and medical professionals. National and international statistics, as stated in the Preface, also support the seriousness of such problems in our society today. In fact, sleep problems are much more common than what is stated in that report because sleep problems were previously not viewed as really serious. Sleep disturbances, including inability to sleep or excessive sleepiness or "sleep attacks," should be taken as seriously as heart attacks or stroke because sleep disturbances have serious consequences affecting the heart,

The ideal sleep requirement is the amount of sleep you need to feel rested, refreshed, and energetic on awakening in the morning and ready to function adequately.

the brain, the circulation, and other systems of the body. This failure to take sleep seriously is a global phenomenon affecting both industrialized and not-so-industrialized nations of the world.

Excessive daytime sleepiness, as a result of inadequate amount of sleep at night due to lifestyle modification or actual sleep disorders such as insomnia or **sleep apnea**, can seriously undercut our productivity and compromise our safety on the road. Many people do not realize that a sleep-deprived driver is as dangerous as a drunk driver. A very common cause of excessive daytime sleepiness or falling asleep at the wheel or at work is sleep apnea (see Question 10), which is a very serious condition but remains underdiagnosed or undiagnosed in thousands of people. Studies performed in Europe, the United States, Israel, and other parts of the world clearly show that the prevalence rate (defined as actual number of patients with sleep apnea present at a particular time in a particular population in a country) for sleep apnea ranges from 1% to 4%. The figures most often quoted are those derived from the Sleep Cohort Study at the University of Wisconsin, which showed that 4% of middle-aged men and 2% of middle-aged women suffer from sleep apnea associated with excessive daytime sleepiness. The Sleep Heart Health Study, another important large-scale study, followed community-dwelling adults for several years and found that 10% of the general population suffers from sleep apnea, and also that most of these people remain undiagnosed. Only a handful of patients are ever referred to a sleep specialist for diagnosis and treatment. Intensive education for both the medical

Sleep apnea

A very serious sleep disturbing condition in which a sleeper stops breathing for at least 10 seconds several times during the night, resulting in interruptions of the sleep cycle.

Sleep Basics

profession and the public is needed to emphasize the presence and seriousness of a variety of disorders, including sleep apnea, affecting our sleep. We are all occupied with two-thirds of our lives during the daytime, neglecting the one-third of our life when we sleep and when a variety of important changes occur in the brain and the body. Many disorders manifest as a result of sleep disturbance. Remember that sleep apnea is much more common than the figures quoted above in certain high-risk populations such as the elderly, obese, and those with a variety of medical (see Question 21) and neurological (see Question 20) disorders. In addition, men in general have a higher prevalence of sleep apnea than women, but postmenopausal women have almost similar rates of sleep apnea as those of men.

5. I was told by my wife that I snore a lot. Why do I snore? Does snoring mean that I have sleep apnea? Or is it just a nuisance?

Snoring is defined as a noisy (mild or loud) resonant breathing during sleep caused by the vibration of the soft tissues in the back of the throat behind the tongue. These soft tissues include the **soft palate** (the soft, muscular tissue in the back of the roof of the mouth), **uvula** (the soft, pear-shaped structure hanging below the soft palate behind the tongue), **tonsils**, back and side walls of the throat, and back of the tongue. Snoring is caused mainly by vibration of the uvula and the soft palate.

Snoring

A noisy sound generated by an obstruction to the free flow of air through the passages at the back of the mouth and nose caused by vibration of the uvula and soft palate during sleep, contributing to reduction of sleep quality.

Soft palate

A soft, muscular tissue in the back of the roof of the mouth.

Uvula

The small piece of soft pear-shaped structure that can be seen dangling down from the soft palate over the back of the tongue.

Tonsils

Areas of lymphoid tissue on either side of the throat.

Snoring can be classified as occasional (mild), frequent (moderate), and severe (very loud, habitual, and frequent). When you sleep, the muscle tone in the back of the throat, including that in the tongue and other muscles in the upper airway passage (through which air goes into the lungs), decreases; an especially marked detrimental absence of muscle tone occurs during the dream stage of sleep (REM). The muscle tone decreases because of decreased signals from the nerve cells or the nerves supplying these muscles. This loss of muscle tone causes the tongue to go toward the back of the throat, slightly narrowing the upper airway and creating turbulence. The turbulence causes vibration, mainly of the uvula and soft palate, which produces snoring. When you lie on your back, the tongue tends to go further back and hence snoring gets worse in this position. In a severe case of snoring, this occurs in all body positions. If you are tired, drink alcohol, or take sleeping medications, snoring becomes worse because the muscle tone is decreased greatly. In the presence of enlarged tonsils, a large and long uvula, or a bulky soft palate, the upper airway passage is narrowed even further, causing loud snoring. Partial obstruction of the nose (because of a cold or allergy that causes swelling of the tissues, for example, or presence of nasal septal deviation) may also contribute to snoring. Snoring affects more men than women, and its prevalence increases with age. An important survey from San Marino, Italy, in the early 1980s found that 60% of men older than 60 and 19% of the overall sample were habitual snorers. Later surveys

Sleep Basics

confirmed the high prevalence of snoring in men. Those who smoke, lie on their back, are obese, and are physically inactive were found to be more likely to snore. Individuals with frequent loud snoring (habitual snorers) are more likely to doze off at the wheel and become involved in a traffic accident.

Mild snoring may be a social nuisance. In contrast, loud, frequent, almost nightly snoring may be the fore-runner of the most serious disorder with severe long- and short-term consequences. That is, it may be the warning sign of something more sinister. Loud snor-ing may repeatedly disturb sleep for brief moments throughout the night. Although the snorer will not remember these brief interruptions in sleep, a record-ing of the electrical recordings of the brain (EEG) will indicate recurrent periods of awakenings. Because the snorer does not get an adequate amount of sleep, he or she is sleep deprived and prone to frequent sleepiness in the daytime. This condition is merely an interme-diate stage before the next stage, when snoring be-comes associated with periodic cessation of breathing throughout the night, signifying a more serious condi-tion than simple snoring. The snorer is now suffering from sleep apnea (see Question 10).

Loud snoring may repeat-edly disturb sleep for brief moments throughout the night.

6. My wife tells me I snore loudly, driving her crazy. I also feel sleepy in the daytime. Should I use a snore guard or see a doctor?

If the snoring is loud enough to drive your spouse crazy, then certainly it is not just a nuisance. In addition, if you feel extremely sleepy in the daytime, then you are experiencing fragmented sleep (repeated brief awakenings at night), which causes daytime sleepiness. This condition may indicate that you are developing sleep apnea (see Question 11). If snoring occurs only when lying on the back, you should try to sleep on either side. If the snoring and daytime sleepiness continue, then you should see a doctor for investigation of possible breathing disorders during sleep.

Numerous advertisements claim cures for snoring and sleep-related breathing disorders. You should, however, be wary of these anti-snoring devices, most of which have no benefit or may reduce the intensity of snoring only temporarily. The best thing to do is to see a physician, preferably a sleep specialist, who can make a positive diagnosis of breathing disorder during sleep early enough to prevent long-term adverse effects.

7. How does sleep affect breathing in a normal person?

During NREM sleep the breathing decreases a little, but during the dream stage of sleep, breathing becomes irregular. The volume of air we breathe also decreases slightly during sleep. As a result, the blood oxygen saturation falls slightly and blood carbon dioxide tension rises a little above the waking level. Respiratory reflexes that maintain normal breathing are also altered, and the arousal responses (intensity of stimulation to wake us up) are altered so that it takes longer to wake us up as we go into the deeper and deeper stages of sleep. As stated above (see Question 5) muscle tone in the back of the throat decreases and the tongue tends to move backward during sleep, narrowing the upper airway and causing partial obstruction to airflow into the lungs. Respiration is, therefore, vulnerable during normal sleep, and a few periods of cessation of breathing may occur, especially at the onset of sleep and during the dream stage of sleep, which do not have any significance in terms of adverse effects.

8. Is snoring related to any physical defect? Can snoring cause any physical illness or memory impairment?

Some of the causes of snoring have been discussed in Question 5. In addition to physical defects in the throat, other defects that may contribute to snoring include a receding chin, a large tongue, and a thick neck. Furthermore, nasal congestion, nasal allergy, and nasal septum defects may promote mouth breathing, which will generate increased resistance in the nasal passages and create turbulence in the back of the throat contributing to the snoring. Snoring is also worse in those who smoke, are obese, consume alcohol, or take sleeping medication (see Question 14). It has also been suggested that loud snoring for a long time may lead to mild swelling of the soft palate and uvula, causing damage to the nerve supplying these structures as a result of repeated vibrations associated with snoring. This theory, however, remains controversial. Early epidemiological studies have cited snoring as a risk factor for high blood pressure, coronary artery disease, or even stroke. But in these studies, most of those patients with snoring probably had sleep apnea (see Question 10), which may cause serious long-term consequences such as high blood pressure, stroke, or coronary artery disease. Some researchers have suggested that snoring may disturb the sleep by repeatedly waking the patient and causing fragmentation of sleep, which may lead to excessive daytime sleepiness and possibly some interference with concentration and attention in the daytime. Early memory impairment in patients with snoring may actually be related to an associated sleep apnea that causes blood oxygen levels to fall repeatedly during sleep at night rather than to snoring itself. There is another way snoring may cause sleep disturbance: snoring, of course, will disturb the bed partner, who may decide to wake up the snoring person briefly or encourage him or her to change positions, thus causing sleep disturbances throughout the night, and the interruption of sleep may cause excessive daytime sleepiness, irritability, and lack of concentration.

9. I am a 65-year-old man falling asleep in the daytime in inappropriate places and under inappropriate circumstances. I have been in one minor car accident and have almost been in two other car accidents because of the excessive sleepiness. Should I see my primary physician or a sleep specialist?

Excessive sleepiness in the daytime that is severe enough to cause or nearly cause car accidents suggests the presence of a serious condition that requires immediate attention. Many older men have such symptoms. One common cause of such symptoms in an older man is sleep apnea (see Question 10). Many patients with this disorder remain undiagnosed and underdiagnosed. It is important to identify the condition early to prevent both short- and long-term adverse consequences. Fortunately, effective treatment is available for most patients suffering from this problem. In order to ensure that this condition is treated, you should see your primary care physician, who may suggest a consultation with a sleep specialist who can evaluate your condition by performing appropriate laboratory tests and suggest optimal treatment.

PART TWO

Sleep Apnea

What is sleep apnea?

Can sleep apnea run in the family?

Can stroke cause sleep apnea or
sleep apnea cause stroke?

More . . .

10. What is sleep apnea?

The cessation of breathing occurring during sleep is called sleep apnea. The term *apnea* is derived from a Greek word meaning "for want of breath." Most people, especially after age 50, stop breathing momentarily a few times during the nighttime sleep. This condition is normal and not a cause for concern. As discussed in Question 7, normal physiological changes in breathing during sleep make us all vulnerable, and there may be a few short periods of apneas without any clinical significance in a normal person. This breathing cessation may occur as many as five times per hour of sleep. To be significant, the breathing must stop for at least ten seconds during sleep. Sometimes breathing may not stop completely but rather be reduced by 30% to 50% of the normal breathing volume, a condition known as **hypopnea**. Like sleep apnea, hypopnea has both short- and long-term adverse effects.

Sleep scientists have defined three types of apneas—upper airway obstructive, central, and mixed types. The most common (and most serious) type is **obstructive sleep apnea (OSA)**. In this type of abnormal breathing during sleep, the passage of inhaled air becomes obstructed in the region of the upper airway, most commonly at the level of the soft palate (see Question 5) but sometimes may occur at multiple sites. Consequently, air does not enter the lungs (the breathing organ responsible for maintaining normal respiration and blood oxygen at an optimal level) and the blood oxygen tends to fall below the normal level. The **diaphragm** (the main muscle of breathing, separating

Hypopnea

The reduction of breathing volume to below the normal level.

Sleep scientists have defined three types of apneas—upper airway obstructive, central, and mixed types.

Obstructive sleep apnea (OSA)

Abnormal breathing during sleep, wherein the passage of inhaled air becomes obstructed in the region of the upper airway.

Diaphragm

The main muscle of breathing, located at the junction of the chest and abdomen.

the lower chest from the upper abdomen) and other chest-wall muscles keep contracting, trying to overcome this obstruction in the upper airway. The brain then sends signals telling the subject to wake up. The person then wakes up with a loud snore. As soon as the individual wakes up, the muscle tone in the upper airway and the tongue returns to normal levels. The tongue moves forward, the obstruction is relieved, and normal breathing resumes. This cycle repeats as soon as the individual returns to sleep.

In a mild case of upper airway obstructive sleep apnea, the cycle of apnea and normal breathing occurs only a few times during the night. In severe cases, the cycle may repeat several hundred times, repeatedly reducing the blood oxygen level throughout the night and disturbing the individual's sleep. Because he or she obtains an inadequate amount of sleep, the person is sleep deprived and sleeps excessively during the daytime in an inappropriate place and under inappropriate circumstances.

In **central sleep apnea (CSA),** the airflow stops at the nose and mouth and the air does not enter the lungs. At the same time, the breathing effort by the diaphragm and other muscles of breathing stops. Central apnea is associated with a number of neurological disorders (see Question 20).

Mixed apnea is characterized by an initial period of central apnea, followed by a period of obstructive apnea. In the most common type of upper airway obstructive

Central sleep apnea (CSA)
Abnormal breathing during sleep, wherein the airflow stops at the nose and mouth and the breathing effort by the diaphragm and other muscles of breathing stops.

Mixed apnea
Abnormal breathing during sleep, characterized by an initial period of central apnea, followed by a period of obstructive apnea.

sleep apnea syndrome, the patient experiences many periods of mixed apneas as well as some central apneas. Sleep apnea is more common in men than women, although its prevalence increases in postmenopausal women. The male hormone testosterone appears to predispose men to sleep apnea whereas the female hormone estrogen acts as a deterrent to sleep apnea.

Researchers have not yet determined why the muscle tone in the upper airway falls excessively in patients with sleep apnea, producing an obstruction in the upper airway. In many patients, the uvula and soft palate are bulky and long, narrowing the airway passage. In children, large tonsils and **adenoids** (lymphoid tissues in the throat behind the nasal passage) narrow the air passage, causing loud snoring and sleep apnea. The nerve cells responsible for maintaining muscle tone in the tongue and other upper airway muscles appear to transmit fewer impulses through the nerves to these tissues. To date, no evidence suggests that most patients with sleep apnea have a structural defect of the nerve cells of the **brain stem** (the lower part of the brain). Of course, neurological disorders (for example, stroke, tumor, trauma, multiple sclerosis) that affect the brain stem or brain may cause sleep apnea in many patients (see Question 20). Why the nerve cells send fewer impulses to the muscles in the back of the throat, including the tongue, is not known and probably is due to functional changes in the nerve cell's core alteration of chemicals (**serotonin, acetylcholine,** noradrenalin) modulating

Adenoids

Lymphoid tissues in the throat behind the nasal passage.

Brain stem

The deeper part in the base of the brain which connects the main brain hemisphere with the spinal cord.

Serotonin

One of the chemicals responsible for inactivation of REM sleep.

Acetylcholine

The main chemical agent causing activation of REM sleep.

these nerve cells. This may also be determined by genetic factors (see Question 12).

Sleep apnea is characterized by a long history of loud snoring, periods when breathing stops repeatedly during sleep at night (witnessed by a bed partner), and recurrent awakenings. The major daytime symptom is excessive sleepiness at inappropriate times and in inappropriate circumstances causing accidents and near-accidents during driving. Long-standing cases of severe sleep apnea may lead to forgetfulness, and in men, impotence. If you have any of these symptoms, it is important to tell your physician, so he or she can make an adequate diagnosis. Although most patients are obese (about 70%) and middle aged or elderly, the condition can also strike thin people and can occur at a younger age. Therefore, close attention should be paid to the important symptom of loud snoring. Repeated cessation of breathing during sleep at night as witnessed by the bed partner and excessive daytime sleepiness for making an adequate diagnosis. Effective treatment will help you avoid long-term adverse effects, including high blood pressure, coronary arterial disease, **heart failure**, irregular heart rhythm, stroke, heart attacks, and impairment of short- and long-term memory. In the literature, several inconsistent figures have been quoted for the prevalence of sleep apnea. Sleep specialists frequently quote the study performed at the University of Wisconsin Sleep Cohort Study (see Question 4). The figures of 2% to 4% given by

Sleep Apnea

Heart failure
The inability of the heart to pump blood adequately to different body regions.

this study include not only the sleep recording abnormalities showing the cessation of breathing but also the daytime symptoms. In the same study, analyzing only the overnight sleep recording, the figures were 24% for men and 9% for women, showing at least five episodes per hour of apneas and hypopneas.

11. What are the clues that I should look for if I think I have sleep apnea?

If you snore loudly almost every night, wake up frequently at night, wake up fighting for breath or suffocating, feel groggy and tired first thing in the morning upon waking up, and feel excessively tired and sleepy during the daytime, you most likely have sleep apnea. You must, therefore, see your family physician, who will refer you to a sleep specialist for an overnight polysomnography study (see Question 27) to confirm the diagnosis and have appropriate treatment. **Table 1** lists some important symptoms of sleep apnea.

12. Can sleep apnea run in the family?

Sleep apnea may sometimes run in the family. In most patients, however, the condition is not familial (see Question 10 regarding sleep apnea). Risk factors (factors that may predispose a person to sleep apnea) include high blood pressure, obesity, alcoholism, and minor abnormalities inside the mouth and face (e.g., long uvula, small upper airway space, receding chin). These risk factors (see **Table 2**) may be inherited, which may explain the high occurrence of sleep apnea in some

TABLE 1 Clues You Should Look for in Suspected Sleep Apnea

- Nighttime Symptoms
  - Long history of loud snoring
  - Choking and gasping during sleep
  - Apneas or cessation of breathing witnessed by the bed partner
  - Excessive movements during sleep causing disarray of bed clothes
  - Excessive sweating at night and increased frequency of urination and sometimes bed wetting, particularly in children
  - Sitting up and waking up with heartburn due to acid reflux
  - Nonrestorative sleep and feeling groggy first thing in the morning upon waking
- Daytime Symptoms
  - Excessive daytime sleepiness and fatigue
  - Dryness of mouth on awakening
  - Morning headache
  - Hyperactivity in children
  - Inattention, forgetfulness, and lack of concentration

TABLE 2 Risk Factors for Sleep Apnea

- Being male
- Menopause
- Increasing age
- Obesity
- Increasing neck size (more than 17 inches in men and more than 16 inches in women)
- Alcohol consumption
- Smoking
- Racial factors (e.g., increasing prevalence in United States among African Americans, Mexican Americans, and Pacific Islanders)

families. There may be genes in the family causing upper airway anatomical abnormalities, abnormal facial features, obesity, and abnormal brain control of breathing, which might increase the risk for developing sleep apnea in such families. However, adequate studies to determine familial incidence have not been undertaken.

13. How are the normal breathing events during sleep changed in sleep apnea?

As stated in Question 7, wakeful breathing changes during sleep, causing a reduced amount of airflow with a mild reduction of blood oxygen saturation and slight increment of the level of carbon dioxide in the blood. When a person with sleep apnea either stops breathing completely or the breathing is markedly reduced in volume, the individual cannot breathe in an adequate amount of oxygen and cannot exhale an efficient amount of carbon dioxide. As a result, the blood oxygen levels fall and the blood carbon dioxide levels rise. The brain senses these alterations in the blood chemistry and sends signals causing an arousal and resumption of breathing. As soon as the person wakes up, the muscle tone in the upper airway and the tongue comes back to the normal waking level, the breathing passage is now open and therefore normal breathing is resumed with a loud snore; sometimes the person will wake up fighting for breath. Depending on the severity of the condition, these changes in the breathing may happen many times throughout the night, interrupting the sleep, which causes nonrestorative sleep interfering with normal daytime functioning. In addition, during resumption of breathing following an apnea, there is an intense stimulation of the **autonomic nervous system** (that part of the nervous system that is not controlled voluntarily but which is needed to continue the vital functions of the body, such as respi-

Autonomic nervous system

The part of the nervous system controlling vital functions of the body such as circulation, respiration and hormone secretion.

ration and circulation) causing a surge of heart rate and blood pressure. This cyclic stimulation of the autonomic nervous system causing transient rise of blood pressure and heart rate during sleep at night may leave the subject with permanent daytime hypertension with all its potentially adverse consequences.

14. Why is snoring or sleep apnea worse after drinking alcohol or taking a sleeping medication?

Consider the mechanisms of snoring and sleep apnea (see Question 5). Snoring or sleep apnea is associated with a reduction of muscle tone in the tongue and other muscles of the throat, which narrows the upper airway space. Alcohol and sleeping medication have a direct depressant effect on these muscles, further reducing the muscle tone and allowing the tongue to move back further, thereby narrowing the upper airway space. In addition, following consumption of alcohol or sleeping medication, stronger stimuli are needed to arouse the brain, therefore prolonging the episodes of apnea or hypopnea. As a result of all these changes, the snoring and sleep apnea worsen.

15. My friend told me that sleep apnea is a serious condition that may cause both short- and long-term serious consequences. Is my friend correct?

Your friend is absolutely correct. Sleep apnea may cause very serious short-term and long-term adverse effects (see **Table 3**). Increasing daytime sleepiness as a

Sleep apnea may cause very serious short-term and long-term adverse effects.

TABLE 3 Adverse Effects of Sleep Apnea

- Short-Term Consequences
  - Increasing daytime sleepiness causing impaired quality of life
  - Increasing traffic accidents
  - Increasing work-related accidents
- Long-Term Consequences
  - Increasing prevalence of high blood pressure in untreated sleep apnea
  - Increasing prevalence of coronary arterial disease
  - Increasing association between sleep apnea and stroke
  - Impairment of memory and cognition (intellectual impairment after long-standing untreated sleep apnea)
  - Increasing prevalence of sleep apnea in heart failure
  - Increasing association with diabetes mellitus

result of waking up frequently throughout the night may cause serious impairment of quality of life. There is a higher incidence of traffic accidents and work-related accidents in sleep apnea patients compared with those who do not have sleep apnea, and these consequences are due to the excessive daytime sleepiness and fatigue. In terms of adverse long-term consequences, there is an increased association between sleep apnea and high blood pressure, stroke, heart disease (irregular heart rhythm and narrowing of the coronary arteries that supply blood to the heart). The question is raised whether sleep apnea by itself or obesity, high blood cholesterol, diabetes mellitus, alcoholism, and smoking (all of which are risk factors for stroke, heart disease, high blood pressure, and sleep apnea) are actually responsible for an increased association of these diseases, and this question remains somewhat controversial. Most investigators, however, believe that sleep apnea is an important risk factor for all of these conditions.

16. I have heard that people with sleep apnea may die suddenly in the middle of the night. Is this true?

Several reports have suggested that sudden death in sleep apnea patients may occur in the middle and late part of the night or in the early hours of the morning. This problem has been reported in patients who suffer from severe sleep apnea, which is associated with repeated prolonged apneas, dangerously low blood oxygen levels, irregular heart rhythms, sleep disruption, and excessive daytime sleepiness. For this reason, it is important to see a physician when symptoms suggest sleep apnea in order to prevent long-term complications affecting the heart, brain, and circulatory system that could potentially elevate one's blood pressure and even cause sudden death.

17. My doctor recently noted that I have high blood pressure. She began treatment but is having difficulty controlling the blood pressure level. I also snore. Can this problem with my blood pressure be due to sleep apnea?

Several studies, including the important Wisconsin Sleep Cohort Study and the Sleep Heart Health Study (see Question 4), have clearly established an association between the presence of sleep apnea and high blood pressure. Approximately 50% of patients with sleep apnea have high blood pressure, whereas 30% of patients with high blood pressure have sleep apnea. Epidemiological studies have also clearly shown the relation between high blood pressure and the degree of sleep apnea (that is, how many times a person stops breathing per hour of sleep). Blood pressure generally drops during sleep, but in patients with sleep apnea, this normal drop in blood pressure is absent. In addition, blood pressure rises periodically and transiently at the end of the apnea and on resumption of normal breathing (see Question 13). These two factors (i.e., absence of the normal fall of blood pressure during sleep at night and periodic rise of blood pressure at the end of apnea) may cause sustained high blood pressure during nighttime, and prospective studies have linked these factors to cardiovascular disorders. In many patients, this nighttime high blood pressure may spill over into the daytime and may become permanently high blood pressure during both the night and daytime. In those with high blood pressure and particularly those who are somewhat resistant to treatment by blood pressure–lowering medications, consideration of the coexistence of sleep apnea must be given because many of these patients have undiagnosed sleep apnea.

18. Can stroke cause sleep apnea or sleep apnea cause stroke?

There is a reciprocal relationship between sleep apnea and stroke. In stroke patients, there is a higher prevalence of sleep apnea. Sleep apnea is also a strong risk factor for developing stroke in the future even after taking into considerations other risk factors such as obesity, high blood pressure, smoking, alcoholism, and diabetes mellitus.

19. What is central apnea and how common is it?

During central apnea the airflow stops at the nose and the mouth and the air does not enter the lungs. At the same time, the breathing effort by the diaphragm (the main muscle of breathing) and other muscles of respiration stops. The most common cause of sleep apnea is upper airway obstructive sleep apnea (see Question 10). In a very small percentage of patients, central apnea is noted. Most commonly, central apnea is associated with neurological disorders including diseases affecting the brain or neuromuscular system as well as with some medical disorders such as heart failure (see Questions 20 and 21). People who ascend to a high altitude (4,000 or more meters above sea level) may also have central apnea as a result of low blood oxygen saturation due to low barometric pressure at high altitude causing stimulation of the breathing. These individuals have periods of apnea followed by hyperventilation, and the apnea cycles repeat, causing repeated awakenings and disturbance of sleep. In some patients, no cause for sleep apnea is found. The patients generally present with excessive daytime sleepiness because of repeated awakenings at night, and some patients may present with insomnia. Central sleep apnea also has similar adverse consequences as those of obstructive sleep apnea (see Question 15). Some types of central apnea respond to medical treatment (e.g., high-altitude sleep apnea), but others require mechanical devices for breathing, such as **continuous positive airway pressure (CPAP)** or bi-level positive airway pressure (see Questions 33–36). Some patients with central apnea may require oxygen inhalation, and recently a special breathing device called assisted servoventilation (ASV) has been used with good results for many patients with central apnea. Some patients with obstructive sleep apnea during **CPAP titration** develop central apnea, and this is called complex sleep apnea. The cause of central apnea is thought to be a fault with the breathing controlling system in the brain.

20. If I have a neurological problem, can I also have sleep apnea?

Most sleep apnea problems are not caused by neurological or other medical disorders. However, if you have a neurological disorder affecting the brain center controlling breathing and the nerves and muscles responsible for maintaining the main breathing and upper airway muscles, you can have sleep apnea. As discussed in Question 18, many patients with stroke have sleep complaints resulting from sleep apnea. An increasing body of evidence taken from several surveys and laboratory studies indicates that sleep apnea and stroke are intimately related. Sleep apnea may adversely affect the long-term outcome of patients with stroke. It is therefore important to make such a diagnosis early because effective treatment is available for this sleep disorder, which may also decrease the risk of having future stroke. Sleep apnea is a well-known complication of **post-polio syndrome**. With this syn-

Continuous positive airway pressure (CPAP)

A remedial therapy involving a small portable machine used to deliver air through the nose to the back of the throat.

CPAP titration

The gradual adjusting of the flow of air until the desired effect is achieved.

Post-polio syndrome

Weakness of arm or leg formerly affected by poliomyelitis, accompanied by paralysis of muscles including those of the previously unaffected extremities, and often breathing difficulties.

drome, there is a history of **poliomyelitis** in childhood or early adult life, accompanied by paralysis of muscles and often breathing difficulties. Years after recovering from the initial illness, the patient may visit a physician complaining of weakness of the previously affected arm or leg muscles plus weakness of the muscles of other previously unaffected limbs. The sleep problem may reflect the past involvement of the nerve cells of the brain that control sleep-wake systems and breathing centers. Many such patients have sleep apnea, which can be documented only by an overnight sleep study (see Question 27). As a result of repeated apneas and reduced ventilation during sleep, they may wake up frequently, which causes interrupted brief sleep and excessive daytime sleepiness. It is important to diagnose the nature of breathing abnormalities because without treatment, these patients may develop long-term adverse consequences associated with sleep apnea (see Question 15). Another important neurological cause for sleep apnea is **Lou Gehrig's disease** (**amyotrophic lateral sclerosis**, or **ALS**). This serious condition is characterized by progressive death of the nerve cells controlling the muscles of the body, including nerve cells regulating breathing. As a result, the patient develops breathing difficulties that worsen during sleep, giving rise to sleep apnea and lowering of blood oxygen saturation. Sleep difficulties in such patients result from repeated episodes of apneas during sleep. The patient also has excessive daytime sleepiness. Although no specific treatment is as yet available to halt the progression of ALS, the patient's quality of life may be considerably improved by treating sleep apnea. Nerve and muscle diseases may also involve

Poliomyelitis

Inflammation of the spinal cord, often called Infantile Paralysis.

Sleep Apnea

Lou Gehrig's disease

Amyotrophic lateral sclerosis (ALS). A serious condition characterized by progressive death of nerve cells controlling muscles of the body.

muscles controlling the breathing, therefore causing sleep apnea with repeated awakenings or repeated arousals during nighttime sleep, leading to excessive daytime sleepiness. Important clues for the possibility of sleep apnea in these patients include excessive daytime sleepiness, breathlessness during the waking period, history of repeated arousals during sleep, and unexplained swelling of the legs due to collection of fluid under the skin for which no apparent cause is found. An overnight sleep study (see Question 27) will detect sleep apnea and any fall of blood oxygen levels during sleep. Treatment of sleep apnea can alleviate sleep problems and prevent long-term complications and improve the quality of life. Many degenerative diseases of the nervous system such as **Parkinson disease (PD)** and Alzheimer's disease may cause sleep apnea. It has been suggested as many as 33% to 53% of patients with Alzheimer's disease suffer from sleep apnea. Alzheimer's disease is the most common cause of dementia. Sleep apnea, by lowering the blood oxygen levels, may cause further nighttime confusion and agitation, aggravating the intensity of the clinical manifestation. Effective treatment of sleep apnea may improve the sleep disturbances as well as confusional agitation in such patients.

Parkinson Disease (PD)

A degenerative disorder of the central nervous system that often impairs the sufferer's motor skills and speech.

Many medical disorders other than neurological diseases may cause sleep apnea.

Emphysema

Excessive stretching of the lungs.

21. Can a medical disorder other than a neurological disorder cause sleep apnea?

Many medical disorders other than neurological diseases may cause sleep apnea. Some important causes include heart failure, bronchial asthma, **emphysema** and chronic obstructive lung disease, allergic rhinitis, and chronic kidney failure. Another common medical disease causing sleep apnea is reduced function of the thyroid gland (located in front of the windpipe in the neck). Normal thyroid function is important for body metabolism. Reduced thyroid function commonly occurs in middle-aged and elderly people and is more common in women than men. If you have reduced thyroid function, you may experience fatigue and constant tiredness, weight gain, slowing down physically and mentally, dryness of the skin, cold sensitivity, and constipation. Cessation of breathing or marked reduction of breathing in this condition may reflect deposition of fatty tissues in the region of upper airway passage, which obstructs airflow to the lungs during sleep. In addition, reduced function of the thyroid gland may affect regulation of the brain centers controlling breathing. You may wake up frequently at night. The insufficient sleep at night leads to excessive sleepiness in the daytime, which could of course be related to the reduced function of the thyroid gland alone without associated sleep apnea. The important thing to remember is that this condition can be effectively treated with thyroid replacement medication, but you may also need special treatment for sleep apnea (see Question 33). Reports in the literature suggest that adequate treatment of sleep apnea can completely relieve sleep disturbance, daytime sleepiness, and other symptoms resulting from reduced thyroid function. It is imperative to consult your family physician, who may refer you to a sleep specialist if you have symptoms suggestive of reduced thyroid function as outlined above to avoid any serious long-term complications.

22. I cannot concentrate well. I become irritable and angry easily and I cannot remember things as well as I used to. I also snore during sleep at night. Can these symptoms be due to sleep apnea?

Sleep scientists in different parts of the world have conducted several studies utilizing clinical history and examination findings as well as neuropsychological tests to document impairment of memory, concentration, and judgment in patients who have been suffering from sleep apnea. Usually the symptoms are noted in patients with moderately severe sleep apnea lasting for a long time. These symptoms may result from repeated lowering of blood oxygen saturation during sleep apnea night after night and repeated sleep disturbance with reduction of total and restorative sleep. As a result of these factors, centers in the brain responsible for memory, judgment, and other higher functions may not be able to function adequately. It has been clearly shown by research studies that memory consolidation takes place during sleep and repeated and chronic lack of oxygen in the brain will impair memory functions. Although somewhat controversial, several studies have shown improvement of the memory and other higher functions after effective treatment with CPAP (see Question 33).

23. I snore and I feel tired all day. On several occasions, I missed my exit on the highway while driving. Can this be due to sleep apnea?

What you are describing suggests brief periods of inattention and possibly you have been dozing off for short periods called **microsleep**. As a result of these brief periods of microsleep, you missed the exit and did not realize that you missed it until you came to the wrong exit. This is, in medical science, known as automatic behavior—that is, doing things automatically and repeatedly without knowing exactly why you are doing it. These symptoms are not specific to sleep apnea but may occur in any condition that causes excessive day-time sleepiness. Therefore, these symptoms may be noted in patients with **narcolepsy** (a disorder charac-terized by an uncontrollable desire to fall asleep, gener-ally seen in young patients) or sometimes in patients who have behaviorally induced insufficient sleep at night causing daytime sleepiness.

Microsleep

Transient periods of NREM stage 1 sleep occuring during sleep deprivation experi-ments.

Narcolepsy

A sleep disorder char-acterized by exces-sive daytime sleepiness.

Sleep Apnea

24. I am a 62-year-old man and rarely suffer from headaches, but recently I noticed that on many mornings I feel groggy on awakening from sleep and have a headache. Can my headache be due to sleep apnea?

Yes, it is very possible your headache is due to sleep apnea, particularly if you also suffer from snoring and if your bed partner notices that you sometimes stop breathing for a few seconds during sleep at night. Not all patients with sleep apnea complain of headache, but a certain proportion of patients do complain of morn-ing headache, which is generally worse within one to two hours after waking up. The cause of this headache is thought to be due to a collection of carbon dioxide in the blood excessively during the episodes of apnea along with lowering of the oxygen saturation in the blood. This happens repeatedly throughout the night, and in a moderate to severe case of sleep apnea, this excessive collection of carbon dioxide in the blood will generally cause dilatation of the blood vessels in the brain, causing the headache. Some studies, however, have shown that some patients with sleep disturbance due to many other causes may have similar headaches, and therefore, these headaches may not be specific to sleep apnea. However, the patients may have other telltale signs and symptoms of sleep apnea (see Question 11). If you snore and complain of headache in the morning, you should see your family physician who may refer you to a sleep specialist or to a sleep laboratory for overnight sleep study (see Question 27) to confirm the diagnosis of sleep apnea for early treatment to avoid any long-term adverse consequences.

PART THREE

Diagnosing Sleep Apnea

How does a sleep specialist diagnose sleep apnea?

What is an overnight sleep study?

What happens if I decline treatment?

More . . .

25. How does a sleep specialist diagnose sleep apnea?

A sleep specialist evaluates your sleep apnea by first taking a history and then performing a complete physical examination. Laboratory tests may then be ordered to confirm the clinical diagnosis. Initially, the physician obtains information regarding your sleep complaints. The history should include not only problems during sleep at night but also symptoms occurring during the day. Many patients complain of repeated arousals throughout the night, sometimes choking or fighting for breath. These patients may also have excessive sleepiness, irritability, or fatigue during the daytime. Some patients complain of dozing off while relaxing and sitting in a chair and watching television or reading a book and also while driving. Therefore, it is important to have information regarding your symptoms during an entire 24-hour period. Your history should cover sleep habits (e.g., bedtime, waking time, number of awakenings during sleep at night); information about drug and alcohol consumption; psychiatric, medical, surgical, and neurological illnesses; history of previous illnesses; and family history. Family history is important because some patients with sleep apnea may have relatives who also suffer from sleep apnea (see Question 12).

Many patients complain of repeated arousals throughout the night, sometimes choking or fighting for breath.

It is also important for the specialist to interview your bed partner or caregiver to evaluate whether you have any breathing abnormalities or snoring during sleep or whether you stop breathing during sleep at night or have unusual movements (many patients with sleep apnea have flailing movements of the limbs immediately upon resumption of breathing after a period of cessation of breathing). Several diagnostic tools are available that are directed at uncovering symptoms of sleep apnea. For example, a questionnaire may ask about snoring, cessation of breathing as noticed by the bed partner, excessive movements during sleep (e.g., movements noticed by the bed partner, or disarray of the bed clothes each morning), daytime fatigue and sleepiness, near-miss accidents during driving, and dozing off while relaxing and watching television. A sleep specialist will ask you to fill out such a questionnaire, which will help in making a tentative diagnosis of sleep apnea. The sleep specialist may also ask questions to assess subjective evidence of excessive sleepiness. One useful tool is the **Epworth Sleepiness Scale**. In this evaluation, you will be asked to rate eight situations on a scale of 0–3, with 3 indicating a situation in which your chances of dozing off are highest. The maximum score is 24, and a score of 10 suggests the presence of excessive sleepiness (see **Table 4**). This scale has been weakly correlated with **multiple sleep latency test (MSLT)** scores (see Question 28), which determine objective evidence of sleepiness.

A physical examination is important to uncover any general medical or neurological illnesses that may be responsible for sleep apnea or for uncovering any risk factors for sleep apnea. After taking a thorough history and completing the physical examination, the sleep specialist will be in a position to suspect whether you have sleep apnea and then can order appropriate labo-

Epworth Sleepiness Scale

A tool used during diagnostic process to assess subjective evidence of sleepiness.

Multiple sleep latency (MSLT)

A scoring system used to determine objective evidence of sleepiness.

TABLE 4   Epworth Sleepiness Scale

Situation	Score*
1. Sitting and reading	—
2. Watching television	—
3. Sitting in a public place (e.g., a theater or a meeting)	—
4. Sitting in car as a passenger for an hour without a break	—
5. Lying down to rest in the afternoon	—
6. Sitting and talking to someone	—
7. Sitting quietly after a lunch without alcohol	—
8. In a car, while stopped for a few minutes in traffic	—

*Scale to determine the total scores: 0 = would never doze; 1 = slight chance of dozing; 2 = moderate chance of dozing; 3 = high chance of dozing.

ratory tests to confirm the suspected diagnosis. Following confirmation of the diagnosis, the sleep specialist will be able to design an appropriate treatment for you.

26. What are some important laboratory tests for evaluating sleep apnea?

Laboratory tests need to be performed to confirm the clinical diagnosis of sleep apnea and to understand the severity of the condition for designing appropriate treatment. Sometimes patients with sleep apnea have frequent abnormal movements such as flailing of the arms and movements of the legs, and therefore laboratory tests are needed to differentiate these movements from parasomnias (abnormal movements and behavior occurring during sleep at night) and seizure disorders because these require different treatment. Of course, laboratory tests are needed to diagnose a primary condition if sleep apnea is thought to result from a general medical or neurological disorder.

The two most important laboratory tests for the diagnosis of sleep apnea are the overnight **polysomnographic study** (see Question 27) and the multiple daytime sleep study (see Question 28). In addition, the maintenance of wakefulness test (see Question 29), which is a variant of the multiple daytime sleep study, may be needed in patients with sleep apnea at a later date to monitor the effect of treatment. This test is particularly important to monitor the effect of continuous positive airway pressure (CPAP) treatment (see Question 34) in airplane pilots and truck or school bus drivers because these occupations involve public safety and it is important to make absolutely certain that their sleep apnea has been effectively treated before they are allowed to drive or fly a plane. In special situations, particularly if seizure disorders or parasomnias are suspected, video-polysomnographic study and prolonged monitoring of brainwave tests (EEG) are needed.

Polysomnographic study

An overnight laboratory test used to diagnose primary sleep problems.

Video-polysomnographic study obtains continuous video monitoring during sleep at night and measures many physiological characteristics (see Question 27) during an overnight sleep study. This test is important to observe any abnormal movements and behaviors that may occur during sleep at night. Movements related to sleep apnea must be differentiated from those related to seizure disorders or parasomnias because these require different treatments.

Video-polysomnographic study

Continuous video monitoring during a sleep study which measures physiological characteristics.

Sometimes, as stated above, patients with sleep apnea may have abnormal movements that may be mistaken for seizure disorders or epilepsy occurring predominantly at night, and it is very important to obtain a prolonged EEG (recording of electrical activity of the brain) during both day and night.

27. What is an overnight sleep study?

During an overnight sleep study, activities from many body systems and organs (physiological characteristics) are recorded. It is a painless procedure that should not cause you any discomfort. No needles are used and you will not receive any electrical shock. You will be connected by many sensors and wires to the equipment that records various activities. A typical recording continuously registers the electrical activities of the brain (EEG), the muscles (electromyogram, or EMG), eye movements (electro-oculogram, or EOG), heart rhythm (electrocardiogram), respiratory pattern, snoring, body position, and blood oxygen saturation during sleep at night. In many laboratories, continuous video monitoring is obtained to correlate any abnormal movements and behavior with the physiological characteristics for a correct diagnosis.

EEG, or electroencephalogram (electrical activities of the brain), is recorded by using several channels of a polygraph. The polygraph is somewhat similar to the "lie detector" machine (polygraph test) used in some court cases. Of course, an overnight study takes place in a sleep laboratory and it records many more physiological characteristics than those studied during lie detector tests.

Electrodes or sensors (small, cup-shaped or flat disks measuring about 5–6 mm) are attached with glue to the scalp (surface of the head) to record EEG. These attachments are painless. The sensors are connected by wires to the amplifiers of the polygraph to amplify the minute currents generated in the brain as a result of difference in electrical potentials between the two areas. The electrical activities generated on the surface of the brain are tiny currents that must be augmented before they can be recognized by the computer. Hence, an amplifier is an essential part of the polygraph.

To record eye movements, surface disks are placed over the upper corner of one eye and the lower corner of the other eye. Recording of eye movements is important to identify different stages, particularly the dream stage of sleep.

Recording of eye movements is important to identify different stages, particularly the dream stage, of sleep.

Electrical activities of the muscles (EMG) are routinely recorded by placing sensors over the chin and outer aspects of the upper legs below the knees bilaterally. Recordings are sometimes made from multiple muscles, particularly in patients who complain of abnormal movements of arms and legs during sleep at night. EEG, EOG, and EMG readings are used to identify the different sleep stages.

In most cases, the pattern of breathing is recorded by using three channels. A sensor is placed over the upper lip below the nose to record airflow through the nose and mouth. A band across the chest and another band across the abdomen register the respiratory effort by recording chest and abdominal exertion during breathing. In the most common type of sleep apnea, called upper airway obstructive sleep apnea, the airflow channels recording activities from sensors placed below the nose show no activity or markedly reduced activity, whereas the channels registering chest and abdominal movements are deflected in opposite directions, indicating obstruction in the upper airway passage in the back of the tongue.

Blood oxygen saturation is recorded throughout the night by using a finger clip. The finger clip registers changes in the color of **hemoglobin** (blood pigment); the color that is shown on the monitor by a number (for example, 90% to 100% in a normal individual) indicates blood oxygen saturation (oxygen is carried in the hemoglobin of the blood). In patients with sleep apnea, the blood saturation falls below 90% when the breathing (airflow) stops. The level of oxygen saturation and the number of times breathing stops or is markedly reduced in volume determines the severity of sleep apnea.

Hemoglobin

Blood pigment, the color of which indicates blood oxygen saturation.

To record snoring, a small microphone is attached over the front of the neck. Body position during sleep is monitored through a position sensor over the shoulder. The degree of sleep apnea is worse when a person lies on his or her back. In a routine overnight recording, one channel is used to record the electrical signal of the heartbeat (electrocardiogram) via sensors or the electrodes placed over the upper chest.

When all the sensors have been placed, the connecting wires are gathered in a bundle and attached to the board next to you. This board is then connected by wires going through the walls or ceiling of the bedroom to the main polygraphic machine or computer in an adjacent room where the technician will monitor the recording and the computer monitors and make the necessary adjustments to obtain the optimal recording. If any of the electrodes (sensors and detectors) are moved, creating artifacts in the recording, the technician will enter your room and reposition the sensor so that artifacts are eliminated. The technician will also watch the video if such a recording is used (most laboratories use such simultaneous video recordings to observe any abnormal movements and behavior during sleep).

You will be asked to come to the laboratory during the evening, usually around 8:00 p.m. The technician will explain the procedure to you and help put you at ease. Making the connections and preparations of the machine and explaining the procedure generally take one to two hours. The technician will then turn the lights off at your approximate bedtime and ask you to get ready to sleep. If you must get up in the middle of the night to visit the bathroom, you can easily disconnect the bundle of wires from the machine and clip it to your pajamas or night wear, then reconnect it again upon returning to bed. In the morning, the technician will come to the room around 6:00 or 7:00 a.m. to turn the lights on, remove the electrodes from your skin, and clean the skin surface. You are then ready to go home unless you are scheduled to have a multiple daytime sleep study (see Question 28).

28. What is a multiple sleep latency test (multiple daytime sleep study)?

Multiple daytime sleep study

A very important test to assess the severity of daytime sleepiness.

A **multiple daytime sleep study**, also known as a multiple sleep latency test (MSLT), is a very important test to assess the severity of daytime sleepiness. The MSLT is an absolute necessity for the diagnosis of narcolepsy, a neurological disorder characterized by the uncontrollable desire to fall asleep in inappropriate places and under inappropriate circumstances beginning in adolescence or at a young age, with or without spells of sudden loss of muscle tone and dropping of things or falling to the ground on emotional excitement, vivid and fearful dreams, often when falling asleep or in the early or late part of the night, and an apparent inability to move when falling asleep or upon awakening lasting for a few minutes. The MSLT is also important to assess the overall severity of sleep apnea and other conditions associated with excessive daytime sleepiness. The test is performed the day after completion of an overnight sleep study. To interpret the significance of the findings in the MSLT correctly, the sleep pattern (the total number of hours of sleep and number of awakenings) and the quality of sleep the night before the test must be known. Any impaired or fragmented sleep during the previous night may cause short **sleep latency** (time to fall asleep) and the appearance of rapid eye movements at sleep onset, thereby introducing confounding factors to the diagnosis of narcolepsy and other disorders causing excessive daytime sleepiness. The MSLT is performed every two hours for four to five recordings, and each recording lasts as long as 20 minutes. The test is conducted two to three hours after the final wakeup in the morning following the all-night study. For example, the test can be performed at 9:00 am, 11:00 am, 1:00 pm, and 3:00 pm. The electrical activities of the brain (EEG), chin muscles (EMG), and eye movements (EOG) are recorded during the 20-minute test. The electrodes or the sensors for these recordings will have been in place from the overnight study. You will be asked to refrain from drinking coffee and smoking in the morning. Following breakfast and explanation of the test, the technician will turn the lights off and ask you to lie down and try to go to sleep. In between the tests, you must stay awake and read, walk around, or watch television, but you must not fall asleep—otherwise, the significance of the findings will be questionable.

The sleep specialist looks for two findings in the MSLT: sleep latency, which is the time it takes you to fall asleep (as determined by the changes in brain wave activity) after lights are turned off, and the presence of sleep onset rapid eye movements (the onset of the dream stage of sleep within 15 minutes of the onset of sleep). Mean sleep latency is then calculated from the values obtained in each nap study. Narcolepsy is strongly suspected if the mean sleep latency is eight minutes or less (indicating excessive sleepiness) and at

Sleep latency

Defined as the time elapsed between lights off and the first onset of any stage of sleep as determined by the changes in brain wave activity.

Diagnosing Sleep Apnea

least two sleep onset rapid eye movements occur in four or five recordings. In sleep apnea, the mean sleep latency may be eight minutes or less, indicating excessive sleepiness, but less than two sleep onset rapid eye movements are observed in four or five nap studies. Any sleep latency of eight minutes or less is considered excessive sleepiness (pathological sleepiness). The mean sleep latency between eight and ten minutes indicates mild sleepiness, and one exhibiting ten minutes is considered normal sleep latency.

29. What is the maintenance of wakefulness test?

The maintenance of wakefulness test, or MWT, is a variant of the MSLT but measures your ability to stay awake. Like the MSLT, this test is also performed at two-hour intervals in a quiet, dark room. You will sit in a chair in a semi-reclined position and be instructed to resist sleep. Four or five such tests are performed, and each one lasts 40 minutes. The test is terminated before 40 minutes if sleep is noted. The mean sleep latency is determined based on these four or five tests. If no sleep is recorded, the mean sleep latency is 40 minutes. The MWT is especially sensitive to determine the efficacy of CPAP treatment in sleep apnea and in assessing the effects of medication treatment in narcolepsy. The MWT is particularly important to determine if it is safe for truck drivers or school bus drivers to drive their vehicles and for pilots to fly their planes. The ability to stay awake in these occupations is critically important. In addition to the MWT, the judgment of the sleep specialist is very important in deciding whether it is safe for these individuals to continue in their occupations.

30. Do I have to have an overnight sleep study in the sleep laboratory, or can I have the test done in my own home?

First and foremost, you must see a sleep specialist, who will take a history and perform a physical examination to make certain there is a high index of suspicion for sleep apnea diagnosis in your case (see Question 11 for sleep apnea symptoms) or if your condition may be associated with another primary sleep disorder or a medical or neurological disorder. You should ideally have the test in the sleep laboratory, even though it may be more convenient for you to have the test done in your home. There are various disadvantages of having the test done in your own home. The greatest problem in the portable monitoring at home or home diagnostic testing (HDT) is the absence of a trained technician to intervene in case of any technical problem with the recording. For example, the electrodes or the sensors may get loose, creating artifacts and thus making it difficult to interpret your recording accurately. If there is a medical emergency (e.g., a sudden and dangerous irregular heart rhythm that may occur in patients with severe sleep apnea associated with very low blood oxygen saturation), there is no trained individual to intervene immediately short of calling 911. Time is of the essence in such a situation, and in a sleep laboratory there are facilities available to handle emergencies. Certain portable units may miss subtle apneic or hypopneic events, thus causing false negative results, which may necessitate repeating the recording in a sleep laboratory. HDT may also cause false positive recordings, resulting in inappropriate treatment. Video recording is generally not available in HDT, and this recording is important because many patients with sleep apnea may have flailing movements that must be differentiated from other abnormal movements and behaviors that may occur during sleep such as seizures. Although the Center for Medicare and Medicaid Services (CMS) recently expanded coverage to include HDT, it is still better to have the testing performed in a sleep laboratory under constant supervision. However, under certain circumstances, unattended portable monitoring or HDT for the diagnosis of sleep apnea may be performed but must be supervised by a sleep medicine specialist and may be used as an alternative to overnight in-lab recording for the diagnosis of sleep apnea patients with a high probability of moderate to severe sleep apnea as determined by the history (see Question 11). The American Academy of Sleep Medicine (AASM) suggested certain guidelines for HDT that are subject to future modifications. HDT is not appropriate for evaluation of patients with associated sleep disorders or neurological or other medical disorders. HDT may be recommended for patients in whom in-laboratory overnight study is not possible (for critically ill patients or patients who cannot be moved to the laboratory) or if there is no sleep laboratory available within a reasonable distance and within a reasonable period of time. An experienced sleep technologist must apply the electrodes or the sensors and explain the procedure to a patient before recommending unattended HDT. A follow-up visit to the sleep clinic must be arranged for discussion of the test results and treatment options. If the test is negative in the presence of high probability of sleep apnea based on your history, or if the test is technically inadequate, you must have an in-laboratory overnight sleep study.

31. What happens if I decline treatment?

There are serious complications and consequences if you remain untreated. Conclusive evidence from various surveys including the National Sleep Foundation's America poll indicates that there is increased risk of motor vehicle accidents associated with untreated sleep apnea. People with untreated apnea are also at increased risk for accidents at work, many of which end in death and severe disability. There is an increased prevalence of sleep apnea among truck drivers, which is a particular concern. Other short-term concerns include excessive sleepiness impairing your quality of life, attention, concentration, and mood. In addition to the short-term consequences, there are many serious long-term complications (see Table 3). Many large-scale scientifically conducted studies have proven that about 50% of patients with sleep apnea will develop chronic hypertension, and 30% of patients with hypertension will have sleep apnea. Several large studies have concluded that even those with mild sleep apnea are at increased risk for developing hypertension, and an intractable hypertension that is difficult to treat may be due to sleep apnea. Several studies have shown that continuous positive airway pressure (CPAP) improves the blood pressure. Strong evidence links sleep apnea

People with untreated apnea are at increased risk of driving accidents as well as accidents at work, many of which end in death and severe disability.

51

with coronary arterial disease with irregular heartbeat, heart failure, and stroke. Many important studies have shown increased mortality with sleep apnea, which is proportional to the propensity of sleep apnea as recorded in the overnight polysomnographic study. There is good evidence of an increased association between sleep apnea and cardiovascular events; however, the evidence against protective effects after CPAP treatment is somewhat weak at present. Irregular heart rhythms in sleep apnea, however, have been shown to respond favorably after CPAP treatment. Finally, there is convincing evidence of increased prevalence of sleep apnea and heart failure, and an increased association between sleep apnea and diabetes mellitus.

32. I have been told by my sleep specialist that I have mild sleep apnea, based on the history and overnight sleep study, but I feel fine. Sometimes I feel a little sleepy in the afternoon and I snore loudly, which does not bother me. Do I still need treatment?

Over time, you may develop more moderate and severe sleep apnea, and have other symptoms—e.g., daytime sleepiness and fatigue, memory impairment, lack of concentration, and, if you are a man, erectile dysfunction. Two important population studies (the Sleep Heart Health Study and the Wisconsin Sleep Cohort Study) have shown that you may develop adverse long-term consequences such as high blood pressure, stroke, diabetes mellitus, heart failure, including coronary arterial disease, and impairment of memory and quality of life. Treatment may prevent these untoward consequences.

PART FOUR

Treating Sleep Apnea

How is sleep apnea treated?

What are some of the problems related
to CPAP therapy?

Who do I consult for the problems related to CPAP?

More . . .

33. How is sleep apnea treated?

Various options are available for treatment of sleep apnea (see **Table 5**), but the best treatment is delivery of positive airway pressure through a mask, a technique called continuous positive airway pressure (CPAP; pronounced "see-pap") therapy (see Question 34). This treatment is effective in 100% of patients when used every night during sleep, but if you find use of CPAP difficult or are intolerant and do not adhere to this treatment, other options should be discussed (see Table 5). You should follow some general measures and lifestyle changes, such as loss of weight if you are overweight by controlling the diet and by regular exercise. The problem with weight-loss programs is that it is very difficult to lose weight, and many patients, after losing weight, start putting weight on again, defeating the purpose. If sufficient weight loss can be achieved, it will definitely improve the sleep apnea and may also help decrease the CPAP titration pressure (see Question 35). In mild cases of sleep apnea, if an obese patient can lose sufficient weight and keep the weight down, then the sleep apnea may be cured; however, adequate studies and long-term follow-up have not been conducted to see if sleep apnea recurs despite sufficient weight loss. You should avoid alcohol in the evening and sleeping pills, which will worsen sleep apnea and snoring (see Question 14). You should also stop smoking because there is a clear relationship between smoking and prevalence of sleep apnea; however, whether stopping smoking will improve the sleep apnea remains to be determined. If you have nasal allergies, you should have appropriate

TABLE 5   Treatment Options in Sleep Apnea

- General Measures
  - Lose weight
  - Avoid alcohol (particularly in the evening) and sleeping medications
  - Stop smoking
  - Avoid supine position (sleeping on the back)
  - Participate in a regular exercise program
  - Treat nasal allergies
- Medications
  - No satisfactory pharmaceutical treatment is available for sleep apnea
- Mask Treatment (Positive Pressure Therapy)
  - Continuous positive airway pressure (CPAP)
  - Bi-level positive airway pressure (BIPAP)
  - Pressure relief CPAP and BIPAP
  - Auto-titrating positive airway pressure (APAP)
  - Oral positive airway pressure (OPAP)
  - Adaptive sero ventilation (ASV)
  - Intermittent positive pressure ventilation (IPPV)
- Surgical Measures
  - Soft palate surgery
  - Uvulopalatalpharyngoplasty (UPP)
  - Laser-assisted uvulopalatalpharyngoplasty (LAUP)
  - Somnoplasty
  - Palatal implant or pillar procedure
  - Nasal surgery
  - Major maxillomandibular surgeries
  - Bariatric surgery
  - Tracheostomy
- Oral Appliances
  - Mandibular advancement device (MAD)
  - Tongue retaining device

---

medications to treat the allergies. Nasal allergies may aggravate the existing sleep apnea, and it is important to treat this condition before beginning CPAP treatment. It is not advisable to sleep in the supine (on the back) position. In this position during sleep, when the muscle tone of the tongue falls, gravity tends to pull the tongue backward, narrowing the airway in the back of the throat, making sleep apnea and snoring worse. Also, in a small subgroup of patients, sleep apnea is noted only while lying on the back; this is called positional apnea. These patients will benefit if they can lie on their sides and not on their back. A tennis or golf ball sewn into the back of pajamas may help patients learn to avoid the supine position; this has often been recommended, but it is somewhat impractical. A full-length wedge pillow may work better than the tennis or golf ball. This type of treatment improves apnea-hypopnea index (number of apneas and hypopneas per hour of sleep) and improves symptoms. One problem in treating positional sleep apnea patients is that this group may become non-positional over time.

Unfortunately, there are no effective medications available to treat problems in the upper airway and, therefore, to treat sleep apnea. In patients with central apnea, particularly high-altitude apnea (see Question 19), medication treatment has been helpful. Medications that treat muscle tone in the tongue and muscles in the back of the throat, and which stimulate breathing, have been tried in patients with upper airway obstructive sleep apnea, the most common type of sleep apnea, but these have not been effective even in cases of mild sleep apnea.

In patients with mild to moderate sleep apnea as judged by the sleep specialist based on the history and physical findings and overnight sleep study, some other options may be tried; however, numerous studies, including the follow-up studies, have shown benefit in about 50% of these patients. Many of these patients again develop snoring and all the other symptoms of sleep apnea after initial improvement following treatment with these other options. Patients with risk factors such as associated high blood pressure or with a history of heart attack or stroke ideally should be treated with CPAP **titration** rather than the other options, because there is a good chance of improvement and correction of abnormal breathing events following CPAP titration, thus minimizing the chance of recurrence of heart attack or stroke in most of these patients.

Options like oral appliances and upper airway surgery may be selected for patients who cannot tolerate CPAP treatment or for those with mild to moderate sleep apnea as defined above without any associated risk factors. The oral appliances include mandibular advancement devices (MAD), which increase the airway space in the back of the throat, thus promoting smooth airflow in and out of the lungs during sleep. If your sleep specialist thinks, after discussion with you about the overnight sleep study results, that you are a candidate for MAD, then he or she will refer you to a dentist who is experienced in using this device for treatment of sleep apnea. Problems with using these devices may include excessive salivation (drooling), dryness of the mouth, **temporomandibular joint** pain, discomfort of the teeth, and facial muscle pain. The mandibular devices have been found to be effective in

Titration

The adjustment made to the CPAP flow generator to deliver optimal pressure level to eliminate sleep disordered breathing events.

Temporomandibular joint

The jaw joint.

about 50% of patients. Another point to remember is that you must have a repeat overnight sleep study as a follow-up in about two to three months after using the device to make certain that your sleep apnea has improved and apnea-hypopnea index has normalized. Another device that has been tried in some patients is called a tongue-retaining device to pull the tongue forward and hold it in a position that will open the airway space in the back of the throat, but this is not effective in most patients, and many patients find it uncomfortable and painful.

Some upper airway surgical procedures are available, such as surgery in the soft palate (tongue-like projection from the roof of the mouth in the back of the throat) and other tissues surrounding the soft palate. This can be performed either by actual surgical resection using a scalpel, by laser technique, or by the reduction of the volume of the soft palate and other tissue surrounding it using radiofrequency technique. These surgeries will cause severe pain in the immediate postoperative period, and there may be some alteration of the voice and some regurgitation of fluids through the nose. It is recommended that a repeat overnight sleep study be performed in those patients who have undergone these surgeries in about three to four months after the procedure (to allow time for healing and getting adjusted) to make certain that significant sleep apnea is not persisting, although in most patients snoring will have been eliminated, causing a false sense of security. Another surgery on the palate is called palatal implant, or **pillar procedure**, in which rods made of polyester material are implanted into the

Pillar procedure

Surgery on the palate in which polyester rods are implanted into the soft palate.

soft palate to prevent the collapse of the palate and narrowing of the upper airway in the back of the throat when the muscle tone falls during sleep. This procedure is helpful in some patients with mild to moderate sleep apnea, but in other patients the problem is not in the region of the palate but in the lower part of the airway, in which case this procedure will not be helpful. Several patients have undergone nasal surgery to remove nasal polyps or to correct nasal septum defects. These surgeries may improve sleep apnea severity to an extent and help the patients tolerate CPAP and adhere to its long-term use, but this surgery does not cure sleep apnea.

If you are extremely obese, measures such as dietary restriction and exercise may not be enough to lose sufficient weight, and you may have to undergo some special procedures such as **bariatric surgery** (e.g., gastric bypass or gastric banding), which may be helpful in achieving weight loss but also have considerable morbidity with long-term side effects and postoperative mortality.

Bariatric surgery
A procedure performed to assist obese patients in achieving weight loss.

If you have severe sleep apnea and are intolerant of CPAP, you may require some major surgical procedures such as maxillo (upper jaw)-mandibular (lower jaw) surgeries. These are major surgeries and are performed in some specialized centers. These procedures carry high morbidity and the usual postoperative mortality for major surgeries. Finally, another option is tracheostomy (making a hole surgically in front of the neck bypassing the obstruction in the upper airway), which was the only option available in the past for sleep apnea treatment before CPAP. Tracheostomy is rarely performed now except for very severe cases of sleep apnea with dangerous arrhythmia (irregular heartbeat) of the heart associated with very low blood oxygen levels in patients intolerant of CPAP.

34. My sleep specialist diagnosed sleep apnea for my daytime sleepiness and snoring and recommended positive airway pressure therapy (PAP). What is PAP and what does this do to my sleep apnea?

Positive airway pressure therapy (PAP) is the delivery of continuous positive airway pressure (CPAP) through the nose using a nasal mask. The **CPAP device** consists of a small, portable machine that can sit on a lamp table at the side of the bed and comprises a **flow generator**, tubing connected to the flow generator delivering room air at a positive pressure, and an interface (e.g., a mask) with head straps and a valve to adjust the pressure of the air delivered through the nose into the back of the throat (see **Figure 1**). A vent hole in the mask prevents rebreathing of expired carbon dioxide.

CPAP effectively treats sleep apnea in almost all patients if it can be used regularly for at least four to six hours per night. You must understand the way CPAP helps you and the benefits of CPAP. CPAP helps you breathe normally. Sleep apnea causes relaxation of muscles in the back of your throat as soon as you fall asleep, which makes the upper airway smaller, as has been proven conclusively by special radiological studies (e.g., magnetic resonance imaging of the upper airway). The

CPAP device

A CPAP device includes a mask, head straps, tubes, and a fan. It reduces snoring and prevents apnea disturbances.

Flow generator

The part of CPAP therapy that delivers room air at a positive pressure.

CPAP is effective in almost all patients if it can be used regularly for at least four to six hours per night.

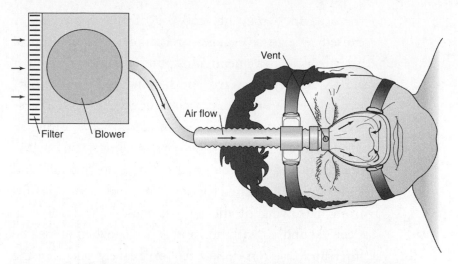

Treating Sleep Apnea

Figure 1 Shows various components of a CPAP device. A blower or a generator produces constant pressure of the room air after passing through a filter. This pressure is then delivered (air flow) via tubing and mask to the upper airway. A vent hole in the mask prevents rebreathing of expired carbon dioxide.

muscle relaxation tends to get worse during the dream stage of sleep, causing the upper airway to collapse, blocking airflow from outside into the lungs. In sleep apnea, outside air is not getting past your upper airway obstruction; if some air gets past the airway, you have hypopnea. In either case, the result is a lowering of blood oxygen saturation and increment of carbon dioxide level. A danger signal is sent to your brain, asking you to wake up by sending arousal signals. As soon as you wake up, the upper airway muscle returns to the normal state and you again breathe normally. As soon as you fall asleep, the muscles of your upper airway relax again, and the cycle repeats. You may have several hundred cycles of no breathing alternating with normal breathing, which results in short- and long-term consequences (see Question 15 and Table 3). CPAP helps by creating positive airway pressure in the back of your throat, which prevents collapse of the upper airway caused by excessive muscle relaxation. The column of air thus acts as a pneumatic splint enlarging the upper airway, mostly sideways, and helping you breathe normally (see **Figure 2**). As a consequence, despite excessive reduction of muscle tone in the throat and tongue, outside air continues to flow into the lungs, you breathe normally, oxygen levels in the blood do not fall, and snoring is eliminated because no turbulence results from narrowing of the air passages. You are able to sleep soundly, without any apnea-related repeated interruptions. You do not feel excessively sleepy in the daytime and, as a result, feel energetic and active and do not complain of fatigue, lack of concentration, and forgetfulness, and, if you are a man, you will notice improvement of your erectile dysfunction.

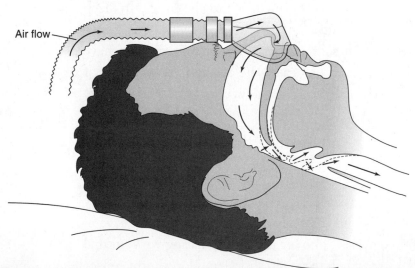

Air flow

Figure 2 Showing airflow (arrows) through tubing and mask to the back of the throat (upper airway) behind the soft palate and the tongue and into the lungs.

You must wear the nasal mask device every night during sleep; otherwise the symptoms will recur. Thus, CPAP treatment is not a cure but gives symptomatic relief. The device may be uncomfortable in the beginning, but approximately 75% of patients become used to it within three weeks.

35. What is CPAP titration and how is it done?

CPAP titration refers to the adjustment made to the CPAP flow generator to deliver optimal pressure level to eliminate sleep-disordered breathing events. CPAP titration is performed during the second night of overnight sleep study in the laboratory after the diagnosis of sleep apnea during the initial overnight recording. Before a sleep specialist can send a prescription for the CPAP equipment, the physician must know the exact positive airway pressure required, which varies from patient to patient, and therefore CPAP therapy needs patient-specific titration. During the titration night study, the technician will attach the electrodes or sensors, as described in Question 27, and monitor your recording looking for apneas, hypopneas, snoring, oxygen saturation and arousals, sleep stages, body position, or other unusual movements and behaviors. The technician begins at the lowest pressure (generally at 4 cm of water) and gradually increases the pressure to completely eliminate apneas and hypopneas, normalize oxygen saturation, and eliminate snoring and repeated awakenings. The technician also will monitor the body position, as sleep apnea gets worse when you are lying on your back or when the pressure needs to be increased. The optimal pressure you need will vary during the night depending on sleep stages and body position. The highest pressure you require during the sleep study becomes the prescription written by the sleep specialist. You will require follow-up visits with the sleep specialist to monitor your progress. In the future, you may need a different pressure depending on weight gain, consumption of alcohol and other medication, as well as other comorbid medical, surgical, or neurological disorders.

36. Where do I get my CPAP equipment?

There are many regional, local, and national home care companies that provide CPAP equipment and related accessories. Your doctor is responsible for prescribing CPAP therapy, including the pressure settings for the machine and the type of interface (mask), but your doctor is not responsible for the equipment itself. Most sleep centers have a list of home care companies, and someone from the sleep center will make arrangements with a home care company for you. The home care company is responsible for supplying the flow generator, the tubing with head gear, and the mask. It will provide a **humidifier** if prescribed by your doctor, and many units have now built-in humidifiers. The home care company will also supply replacement filters for the flow generator and replacement masks when needed. Most of the time, someone from the home care company will contact you to come to your house with the unit and explain how it works and how to take care of the unit (see **Figure 5**). This person will

Humidifier

A device that adds humidity to breathed air to prevent drying of nasal passages.

show you basic procedures like turning the machine on and off, changing the filter, changing the tubing, and putting on your mask. Some home care companies will mail the unit along with the instructions on how to use it. However, it is best for someone to come to your house to instruct you personally, and you should insist on that. If you have any problems, you should contact the sleep center where your overnight sleep study and titration were performed. You should ask the home care company to show you a variety of CPAP units and different types of masks (see **Figures 3** and **4**). Before using the unit, you must be comfortable wearing the

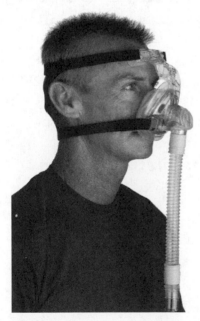

Figure 3   One type of mask available.

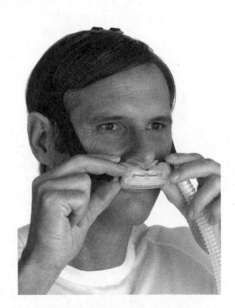

Figure 4   One type of mask available.

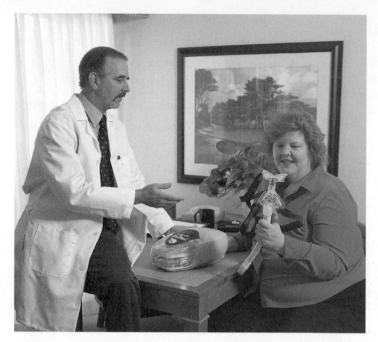

Figure 5   A healthcare provider explaining proper use and care of a PAP machine and mask.

mask and must be knowledgeable about how the unit operates and whom to contact in case of problems with the unit.

37. Are there positive pressure devices other than CPAP?

There are several other types of positive pressure devices that may be needed for certain individuals and for certain types of sleep apnea—e.g., central apnea or periodic breathing, which is a type of central apnea that is found in patients with heart failure or neurological disorders. Table 5 lists all the positive airway pressure devices available for treating sleep apnea. The most common device used is CPAP for treating upper airway obstructive sleep apnea, the most common type of sleep apnea.

Some individuals may complain of difficulty during titration when the same pressure is delivered during inhalation and **expiration** (expelling the air). For such patients, the CPAP device can be adjusted so that it delivers higher-pressure air during inhalation and lower-pressure air during expiration, causing bi-level delivery of positive airway pressure. **Bi-level therapy** may also be used for patients with persistent nasal mask leaks during CPAP titration as well as for patients with comorbid lung disease or chest wall diseases, neuromuscular disorders, or central apnea (see Question 19) unresponsive to CPAP. Recently, devices with pressure relief technology have been introduced for patients who find it very uncomfortable to use either CPAP or even bi-level therapy during titration. In these devices, the pressure during beginning of exhalation only is reduced, and this can be performed both during CPAP and bi-level therapy titration.

Auto-titrating positive airway pressure devices (APAP) do not need manual titration by a technologist, but the computer is programmed to detect abnormal breathing events (apneas, hypopneas, limitation of airflow) and snoring, which are interpreted by a central processing unit (CPU) of the computer based on certain algorithms that vary from one manufacturer to another.

Expiration
Exhaling air during breathing.

Bi-level therapy
A CPAP device that can be adjusted so that it delivers higher-pressure air during inhalation and lower-pressure air during expiration.

The theoretical advantage of APAP is that the pressure is adjusted throughout the night so that the patient does not need to have the same fixed pressure as is used in CPAP through different stages of sleep. Some patients may find constant fixed pressure uncomfortable, especially those who complain of air swallowing and abdominal bloating after CPAP therapy. Generally, the APAP uses overall slightly less (about 2 cm of water) pressure than the fixed CPAP pressure. The improvement in symptoms and correction of the breathing events are similar in both types, but there is no difference in terms of long-term **adherence** (compliance). APAP has certain disadvantages, which include higher cost of the unit, which is, however, compensated by the fact that APAP is an unattended in-home titration and therefore the total cost may be reduced. The other disadvantage of APAP is that different manufacturers use different algorithms, and therefore the findings from one cannot be extrapolated to the other, and cannot be compared. Furthermore, many APAP devices use snoring as an algorithm to detect upper airway obstruction and hence cannot be used in patients who do not snore (e.g., those who have had post–upper airway surgery and a very small number of sleep apnea patients). APAP also cannot differentiate between central and obstructive apneas, and it cannot be used in patients with sleep apnea resulting from neuromuscular diseases, chronic lung diseases, neurological disorders, or heart failure.

Another recently introduced device that has been an alternative to nasal or full-face mask is the oral positive

Adherence

A willingness to continue with long-term therapy.

airway pressure (OPAP) appliance, which many patients unable to tolerate CPAP or bi-level therapy find useful. This device does not require head gear; it bypasses the nose, and therefore some people, especially those with nasal congestion, find this more comfortable. However, air leak through the nose is a problem, and the utility of this device has not yet been established.

Adaptive servoventilation (ASV) is a new technique of PAP therapy for patients with central apneas associated with heart failure and other causes of central apnea without any identifiable cause. An ASV device provides pressure support to maintain the volume of air breathed by the patient so that there is no hyperventilation, which causes periodically recurring apneas and hyperventilation. This system has been found to be useful in patients with central apneas who do not respond to CPAP or bi-level therapy with or without oxygen inhalation.

Intermittent positive pressure ventilation (IPPV) is a special type of positive pressure ventilator required to support the breathing in patients with neuromuscular disorders (e.g., muscle diseases, Lou Gehrig's disease, post-polio patients) and other neurological disorders. Most patients with sleep apnea do not need this system.

38. Does CPAP help central apnea?

CPAP treatment helps certain patients with central apnea where there is an associated component of obstructive apnea, and CPAP along with the delivery

CPAP treatment helps certain patients with central apnea where there is an associated component of obstructive apnea.

of supplemental oxygen through the CPAP unit may help certain patients with central apnea with associated heart failure. Generally, these patients require bilevel therapy with or without supplemental oxygen or ASV (see Question 37).

39. I am symptom free now after using the CPAP. Can I stop CPAP? How long do I have to use it?

It will be a serious mistake for you to stop using the CPAP because you are symptom free. The purpose of CPAP is to prevent obstruction in the back of your throat so that you can breathe normally, and in a way it is a symptomatic and not a curative treatment. Therefore, if you stop using CPAP, all your breathing problems will recur and you will begin to have symptoms along with all the adverse short- and long-term consequences (see Question 15). Sleep apnea is a lifelong condition like diabetes mellitus. Therefore, you have to continue to use the CPAP for your sleep apnea, just like a diabetic patient needs to use anti-diabetic medication or insulin injections indefinitely.

40. What are some of the problems related to CPAP therapy?

CPAP therapy may cause several problems, some of which are common and others which are very rare, in certain patients, but fortunately most of these side effects can be resolved by appropriate measures. **Table 6** lists some common side effects associated with CPAP therapy. Most patients find it somewhat

TABLE 6   Common Side Effects of CPAP Therapy

- Mask and Head Gear (Strap)–Related Problems
  - Skin abrasion or skin rash
  - Chafing of the bridge of the nose
  - Air leaks around the mask causing eye irritation and sometimes conjunctivitis
  - Unintentional removal of mask
- Pressure-Related Problems
  - Difficulty exhaling
  - Uncomfortable feeling
  - Difficulty initiating or maintaining sleep (sleep onset or maintenance—insomnia) and repeated awakenings
  - Air swallowing and abdominal distension
  - Chest discomfort
  - Sensation of suffocation
  - Nasal sinus discomfort
  - Mouth leaks
- Nose-Related Problems
  - Running of the nose and congestion
  - Dryness and stuffiness of the nose
  - Bleeding from the nose
- Miscellaneous Problems
  - Noise of the device
  - Cumbersome, inconvenient, and may cuase loss of intimacy
  - Bed partner's intolerance of the device
  - Claustrophobia

uncomfortable to wear the mask and sleep with it on the face. The mask needs adjustments to either tighten or loosen the straps to prevent air leaks around the mouth and to prevent abrasion on the bridge of the nose or irritation of the eyes due to air leaks. It is essential to treat air leaks because they will make the CPAP therapy less effective, as you will not get the correct pressure to relieve the obstruction in the back of the throat, and therefore apneas and hypopneas will

Treating Sleep Apnea

persist. Most people get used to the mask quickly. There is a considerable individual variation in acceptance of the mask. Some people suffer from side effects related to mask and head gear strap, pressure-related side effects, nose-related problems, and miscellaneous other side effects (see Table 6). The mask-related side effects include skin abrasion or skin rash due to the tight-fitting mask cutting into or irritating the skin, chafing of the bridge of the nose due to pressure of the mask, and air leaks around the mask causing eye irritations and sometimes conjunctivitis and unintentional removal of the mask. Positive pressure–related side effects include difficulty exhaling because of the high pressure, an uncomfortable feeling, difficulty initiating or maintaining sleep causing sleep onset or maintenance insomnia with repeated awakenings, air swallowing with bloating and distended feeling of the abdomen, chest and nasal sinus discomfort, mouth leaks, and a sensation of suffocation. The chest discomfort is related to positive pressure during exhalation causing stretching of the chest wall muscle and other structures, giving rise to a sensation of chest wall problems that may persist even on awakening.

Most people breathe through the nose, and CPAP therapy may sometimes cause nose-related problems, which include running from the nose and congestion, dryness and stuffiness of the nose, and sometimes even bleeding from the nose. The nose normally has two functions: breathing (unless you are a mouth breather) and conditioning of the inspired air (adding moisture).

The air we breathe in is cooler than the air we breathe out. Mouth leaks during CPAP therapy are common and are mostly responsible for nasal symptoms. If you suffer from nasal allergies or sinus infection, then of course you will have nasal symptoms during CPAP therapy with or without mouth leaks. Let me explain how mouth leaks cause nasal symptoms. When there are mouth leaks of air during CPAP therapy, there is increasing flow of air through the nose during inspiration, causing increased resistance to airflow. An increase in nasal resistance encourages mouth breathing, and mouth breathing during CPAP therapy causes increasing nasal resistance, thus creating a vicious circle. This increased airflow and resistance lead to cooling and drying of the nasal route, resulting in compensatory dilation of the blood vessels of the nose, causing congestion and running of the nose. The more the mouth leaks, the more nasal airflow. Nasal symptoms during CPAP therapy will cause suboptimal treatment because of failure to deliver adequate positive pressure to overcome upper airway obstruction in the back of the throat.

Miscellaneous side effects include noise of the device, although the modern flow generators are much quieter than the first-generation units used several years ago. Some patients complain that the device is cumbersome and inconvenient to use, and they feel this prevents them from being intimate with their bed partner. The other problems are bed partner intolerance of the device and claustrophobia.

See **Table 7** for some solutions to common CPAP side effects.

TABLE 7 Solutions for Some CPAP-Related Problems

Problems	Solutions
• Nasal congestion, running from the nose, or dryness	• Use heated humidification. • Use nasal spray. • Treat mouth leaks. • Treat nasal allergies. • Use full face mask.
• Mouth leaks	• Use heated humidification. • Use chin strap (not a good alternative). • Use full face mask.
• Mask leaks	• Make sure mask fits properly, and if necessary change mask. It is also good to have an appointment with the adherence (compliance) or mask clinic at the sleep center.
• Mask discomfort	• The mask may be the wrong size or the wrong mask; contact the home care unit or the sleep center clinic.
• Dry mouth	• Use heated humidifier. • Treat mask leaks. • Treat nasal symptoms. • Find the correct mask to prevent air leaks. • Use full face mask if all else fails.
• Still snoring on CPAP	• There may be inadequate pressure and you may need to increase the CPAP pressure setting. • Consider other factors (e.g., alcohol consumption, sleeping medications). • Lose weight.
• Irritation of the skin of the face and eyes due to air leaks	• Attend to proper mask fitting to prevent air leaks.
• Chafing of the bridge of the nose	• Loosen the head gear slightly and use a soft pad over the bridge of the nose if needed. If these measures fail, a different type of mask may be used with benefit.

41. My sleep specialist told me that there is an initial period of adjustment to get used to the CPAP therapy. What is this adjustment?

The initial period of adjustment may last from four to six weeks. There may be a psychological adjustment for both you and your spouse. You may have psychological worries about the relationship with your bed partner and a feeling of invalidity. Your bed partner may also be psychologically disturbed by the prospect of sleeping with a person who is wearing a mask and head gear resembling a man or woman from outer space. A thoughtful discussion with your bed partner will allay such psychological fears. It is very important to understand the various problems and how to correct them as well as the advantages of having CPAP therapy. You need motivation, and sometimes a sleep apnea support group may help by emphasizing that "you are not alone" with this problem. Your mask may need adjustment if it is too tight or too loose. You need to get used to the head gear and look for air leaks around the mask and the mouth. You have to get used to the soft noise generated by air leaks through the vent (to prevent rebreathing and carbon dioxide retention and intoxication). You must persist and try to get used to wearing the mask; don't give up! Think of all the serious consequences (see Table 3) of not using CPAP every night (see Question 15).

There may be a psychological adjustment for both you and your spouse.

42. Who do I consult for the problems related to CPAP?

First you contact your home health care company; the person there may be able to take care of most of the problems and suggest solutions. You should also contact the sleep center where your study was done. The personnel at the sleep center and the sleep specialist will be able to suggest solutions to your problem. Most sleep centers have special clinics run by the center personnel to demonstrate different types of masks so that you can find out which one is most comfortable for you. The personnel will also be able to explain to you several side effects and how to resolve them as well as how to take care of the CPAP unit.

43. How do I take care of mask-related problems?

A properly fitted mask is the key to success.

There are several mask-related problems (see Question 40 and Tables 6 and 7). A properly fitted mask is the key to success. Many types of masks are available to choose from (see Figures 3, 4, and 5), and you should try all of them to find the one which suits you best. Do not overtighten the mask nor keep it too loose; both will cause air leaks. To prevent chafing of the bridge of the nose, loosen the head gear slightly and use a soft pad over the bridge of the nose. If these measures fail, try a different type of mask. You have choices: there has been considerable improvement with masks designed by different companies, and a variety of masks that are now available, including some with nasal pillows or prongs that fit inside the nostrils.

However, the problem with nasal pillows is that they are liable to be displaced if you turn and try to sleep on your side. Other problems include mouth leaks, swelling, and congestion inside the nostrils. You must also clean the mask daily. Also, to prevent eye irritation, you may have to use an eye patch.

44. How do I take care of pressure-related problems?

There are several solutions to pressure-related problems (see Question 40 and Tables 6 and 7). First, you may use pressure ramp, where the machine is set up at lower pressure for the first 15 to 20 minutes, which is the time you may take to fall asleep. The pressure will then gradually build up to your set pressure. This technique will avoid the uncomfortable feeling of using a mask while you are awake, trying to get to sleep. If you feel you are getting too much pressure, consult your sleep specialist, who may see you in the clinic or suggest that the pressure be lowered somewhat, sending a prescription to the home care company, which will reduce the pressure to the appropriate level.

If you find the CPAP uncomfortable with the same pressure during inspiration and exhalation, you may benefit from BI-PAP, where lower pressure is used during exhalation. Also, you may get relief from using a device that lowers the initial pressure of exhalation, making it more comfortable. You may also contact your home care company to check the pressure to make sure that the setting is correct. If you feel that you are not getting enough air or you are getting a sense of suffocation, check for mask leaks. If you use a ramp feature, contact your home care company to increase the starting ramp pressure. If after following all the above steps you are still intolerant, you should consider other options such as a mandibular advancement device or throat surgeries (see Question 33).

45. How do I take care of problems related to the nose?

Many patients have problems related to the nose (see Question 40 and Tables 6 and 7). For nasal problems, the best suggestion is to use humidification, particularly a heated humidifier. Humidification is especially important for those with nose bleeding or with a history of nose bleeding. The mechanism of how humidified air helps nasal symptoms is described in Question 40. Humidification, especially heated rather than cold-air humidifiers, which add little humidity, will disrupt the vicious circle of increased nasal resistance and mouth leaks and help relieve the nasal symptoms. The personnel from the home care company have already set the temperature in the heated humidifier at a certain level. However, sometimes the air flowing between the humidifier and the mask cools rapidly, causing condensation inside the tube connecting the humidifier to the mask. This problem can be resolved by reducing the humidifier temperature. If humidification does not resolve the problems, consult your sleep specialist, who may suggest that you use nasal sprays such as saline, nasal decongestant, or some topical

nasal steroids or aerosols, particularly if you have allergic nasal discharges. If the problems persist, you must
consult an ear, nose, and throat physician to correct
any problems inside the nostrils.

46. How do I take care of other (miscellaneous) problems?

If the noise is bothersome, particularly for your bed
partner, you may ask the home care company to give
you longer tubing so that the unit can be placed farther
away from the bed. Sometimes a white noise machine
that produces continuous background sound such as
ripples of ocean waves may be helpful.

Some patients suffer from claustrophobia and are
afraid to use the mask, as they have a sense of not
being able to breathe in or breathe out, and feel a sense
of suffocation and a fear of impending death. If you
have these feelings, contact your sleep center; the clinic
personnel can explain the technique of desensitization.
You should try to put the mask on while you are awake
and try getting used to low pressure initially, and then
gradually increase the pressure. Later, you can put the
mask on while lying down in bed and finally during
sleep. Some patients gradually get desensitized and are
able to use it. This gradual increase of use in terms of
hours and gradual increase of pressure may take several
days to achieve a satisfactory result. You can also use a
different style of mask if that allays the fear. Some
patients may do well using OPAP (see Question 37) if
the device fits only the mouth and does not cover the

If the problems persist, you must consult an ear, nose, and throat physician to correct any problems inside the nostrils.

nose or the whole face. If all these measures fail, you should consider other options such as an oral appliance or throat surgery.

47. My mouth and throat feel dry when I wake up in the morning. What can I do about it?

As stated in Question 40, the dryness is due to mouth leaks, which are very common during CPAP therapy and are responsible for nasal symptoms. Humidification, by preventing the vicious circle of nasal symptoms and mouth leaks, will correct the problems in many patients. If you are a habitual mouth breather and if the humidification does not help, the best choice is to use a full face mask covering the nose and the mouth. Several types of full face masks are available. Some patients, however, become claustrophobic with these devices. If you are claustrophobic, a chin strap to keep the mouth closed along with the nasal mask may help. Most of the time, however, the chin strap does not work. A full face mask prevents increased nasal airflow and resistance, thereby preventing mouth leaks.

Humidification, by preventing the vicious circle of nasal symptoms and mouth leaks, will correct the problems in many patients.

48. My friend told me that if you use a humidifier, bacteria may grow inside the water container, which may cause respiratory infection. Is this true?

No cases have been reported so far of upper respiratory infection caused by this mechanism. There are several reasons for this. The upper airway acts as a defense against infection, the temperature of the humidifier is a deterrent to bacterial growth, and the molecules of water generated by the heated humidifier are too small to carry bacteria. However, because of the remote possibility of such infection, you should use sterile, distilled water.

49. I wake up in the morning and often find that my mask is off my face. It seems that I remove it subconsciously. Can I do something about it?

The first thing is to find out why you take the mask off. It may be that you are not very comfortable with the mask, and therefore you should make sure the mask fits correctly (see Question 43). It is probably a good idea to make an appointment with the sleep clinic to find out if the mask is of appropriate size and fitting properly. Changing to a different type of mask might solve the problem. Another thing to look for is if you have any nasal symptoms that interfere with breathing through the nose and thus cause you to take the mask off. Any nasal symptoms should be treated (see Question 45). You should try hard to wear the mask, and if you keep trying, you may get used to it and will not inadvertently remove it. Another thing that may have happened is that you may have gone to the bathroom and removed the mask but did not put it on when you came back to bed. Sometimes if you are in deep, slow-wave sleep, a state of partial arousal causing a transient confusional episode may occur during which you might inadvertently remove the mask. If you try to adhere and motivate yourself to use the mask, you may gradually notice that your sleep

You should try hard to wear the mask, and if you keep trying, you may get used to it and will not inadvertently remove it.

improves. Remember that wearing the mask in the early hours of the morning is extremely important, as at that period the dream stage of sleep is most intense. Sleep apnea gets worse with marked lowering of blood oxygen saturation, which will cause long-term adverse consequences, as discussed in Question 15.

PART FIVE

Living with Sleep Apnea

Should I take my CPAP unit with me when I travel?

Do I need a regular follow-up visit
with my sleep specialist?

How do I take care of my CPAP equipment?

More ...

50. I was told by a friend that about 25% of patients do not use their CPAP long term. Why is this?

Your friend is correct that many patients fail to accept or adhere to using the CPAP for long-term use. I will try to explain the reasons and provide some solutions to these problems. Let me explain what I mean by acceptance and adherence. Acceptance can be defined as willingness to start treatment with CPAP, and in various studies the rate of acceptance has varied from 60% to 90%. There are several reasons for this: difficulty falling asleep, frequent awakenings during sleep at night, and discomfort with the mask. The solution is to pay attention to the mask discomfort, mouth leaks, and nasal symptoms, as discussed in Questions 43 and 45.

Adherence (previously known as compliance) can be defined as willingness to continue with long-term CPAP therapy. Studies have shown a wide variation in the rate of adherence, and as many as 12% to 25% of patients discontinue using CPAP therapy by three years. Some studies have found that 40% to 60% of patients used CPAP for four hours or more per night. This percentage has shown improvement after intensive education and discussion of the methods to increase acceptance and adherence. Education, not only of the patient but also of the bed partner, is important. Other measures to increase adherence include attention to the mask fitting and comfort, treatment of the nasal symptoms, use of heated humidification, and attention to the other side effects. Regular clinic follow-up visits and regular contact even by

telephone with the sleep specialist, home care personnel, or sleep center personnel are essential for good
outcome in this respect. The pattern of CPAP use is
usually established in the first two weeks, and therefore
early intervention is very important. It has been noted
from various studies that certain patients accept and
adhere to CPAP therapy better than others. Most
patients with severe sleep apnea associated with severe
daytime sleepiness, those who referred themselves
(self-referred) to the sleep clinic because of the severity
of symptoms, and those who have better coping strate-
gies are the ones who will accept and adhere to CPAP
use for the long term. These patients perceive the
benefit of CPAP therapy more readily than others.
Another important measure is for the sleep specialist to
objectively monitor your adherence to the CPAP use.
Many CPAP units are now fitted with "smart cards"
with memory showing hours of use of the machine at
the correct pressure and the hours the machine was
turned on. It is important to pay attention to hours
actually used with correct pressure rather than the
hours the machine is turned on; some patients may
turn the machine on but may not use it continually.

51. I am going to have surgery. Do I need to tell my surgeon about my sleep apnea and CPAP therapy?

You must tell your surgeon as well as the person giving
anesthesia for your surgery about your sleep apnea and
CPAP therapy. A patient with sleep apnea is liable to
have more complications and consequences than one

The pattern of CPAP use is usually estab-lished in the first two weeks, and therefore early intervention is very impor-tant.

Living with Sleep Apnea

without sleep apnea after surgery and after administration of general anesthetics. The anesthetics used as well as the painkilling medications and sedatives used during the operation and the postoperative period will suppress the muscle tone in the upper airway, causing more breathing problems, and some of the agents, particularly the morphine group of drugs and the anesthetics, will have an adverse effect on the breathing centers in the brain, causing depression of respiration. The person giving the anesthesia (anesthesiologist) will take appropriate measures to prevent this serious complication and therefore must be aware of your sleep apnea. It has also been shown in several studies that postoperative complications are worse after major surgery for those with sleep apnea than those without sleep apnea. Also, in the postoperative period, your sleep pattern may change. For example, the dream stage of sleep after recovering from the effects of anesthesia may increase, and during this stage, the breathing even gets worse, causing further lowering of the blood oxygen saturation. You must also take your CPAP unit to the hospital, where it should be tested for electrical safety and cleanliness to make sure that there are no bacterial contaminants in the unit. You must use CPAP before and after surgery so that you do not miss using it for even one night to avoid reemergence of symptoms. These measures will minimize postoperative complications.

52. Should I take my CPAP unit with me when I travel, including foreign travel?

Yes, you must take your unit when you travel on vacation or business either within or outside the United States. Various studies have shown that if you do not use the unit, even for one night, your symptoms will return and you will be liable to develop all those long-term adverse circumstances discussed in Question 15. You must take the equipment in a carrying case, and you must not check this case as baggage because it is liable to be damaged. Airport security personnel are generally knowledgeable about CPAP machines and they will pass the check point, but you should be prepared to open the case and show the security personnel the CPAP equipment. You should also be sure to keep a copy of the manual as well as the prescription showing the correct pressure in case you have some problems with the machine while you are away from your home. The sleep center or sleep specialist in the place you are visiting may be able to help you find a new unit through a respiratory care company so that you do not spend a single night without using a CPAP. You should also bring a long extension cord and an extra fuse. If you travel to a foreign country, the electrical requirements may be different from those in the United States. The electrical circuits in the United States operate at 110 volts and 60 cycles per second. However, electrical circuits in many overseas countries use 220 volts and 50 cycles per second. Therefore, before foreign travel you should acquire an appropriate converter and adapter. Some modern machines are fitted with internal automatic converters that will automatically adjust. You should also be aware of the effect of high altitude. If you travel to a place that is more than 5,000 feet above sea level, you will need adjustment of the CPAP pressure. At high altitudes, the barometric pressure falls and you may need to increase your CPAP pressure setting in order to continue to get the adequate amount of air to keep the upper airway passages open to avoid snoring and apneic events during sleep. Your home care personnel can give you instructions about adjustment of the pressure, or someone from the home care company may come to your home to adjust the pressure. However, you must remember to change the pressure back to the original settings when you return home.

53. Do I need a regular follow-up visit with my sleep specialist? If so, for how long?

Regular follow-up care at the sleep clinic is very important. Remember that sleep apnea is a lifelong condition as far as we know today; hence, it must be considered a chronic illness, and like any other chronic illness (e.g., diabetes mellitus, high blood pressure) continuous monitoring and treatment are required. Active follow-up care is a key to adherence (see Question 50), and adherence is the key to success to preventing long-term adverse consequences of sleep apnea. Many studies and surveys have conclusively proven this point. Follow-up care is important to make sure that your equipment is working properly and you remain symptom free. Your symptoms may reappear, for example, due to the fact that the equipment is not functioning properly or the mask is not fitting properly, because you have either gained or lost weight, or because you are on certain medications for other medical or neurological conditions that might make sleep apnea worse. It is important to assess your overall condition at periodic visits, otherwise you are liable to have all those adverse long-term consequences.

54. Despite using my CPAP regularly on a nightly basis, I have persistent sleepiness in the daytime. Why is this, and what should I do?

If your persistent sleepiness is due to persistent sleep apnea, you are liable to have long-term adverse consequences as discussed in Question 15. Persistent sleep apnea may be due to low nightly CPAP use (not using it every night or using it for only a few hours and not at least four to six hours per night) or mask and mouth leaks. If you do not have persistent sleep apnea as proven by a repeat overnight polysomnography study, and you still have persistent sleepiness despite using CPAP regularly on a nightly basis for at least four to six hours, you should then consider several other factors to explain the sleepiness. First, the diagnosis may have been incorrect in the first place and perhaps you

Follow-up care is important to make sure that your equipment is working properly and you remain symptom free.

Living with Sleep Apnea

should be reassessed. Your CPAP titration final pressure may have been inadequate or you may have gained weight. You may have other new medical or neurological disorders or another primary sleep disorder (e.g., narcolepsy is sometimes noted with sleep apnea). You may be now suffering from depression causing excessive daytime sleepiness. It has been shown that the prevalence of depression and insomnia may be somewhat increased in patients with sleep apnea. Another cause may be use of alcohol or sleep medication or other medications you need for treating your associated medical disorders. Finally, after excluding all these factors, a small subgroup of patients with sleep apnea will have residual or persistent sleepiness despite using the equipment regularly for a sufficient amount of time. The cause of this is not known, but it has been suggested that there may be some unknown effect on the brain as a result of lowering of the blood oxygen levels repeatedly during sleep apnea for a long time. After exclusion of all these factors discussed above for persistent sleepiness, sleep specialists will sometimes use a stimulant medication in addition to CPAP therapy to correct the persistent daytime sleepiness. The two drugs approved for such treatment are modafinil or armodafinil, novel wake promoting agents, which have fewer side effects than the traditional stimulants. These are prescription medications, and your sleep specialist is the best person to decide if you may benefit from one of these drugs. Your sleep physician will also discuss the side effects and drug-drug interactions with you.

55. If my sleepiness improves after taking stimulant medication, why do I have to keep using my CPAP?

Stimulant medication is used for a specific symptom of daytime sleepiness that is not related to sleep apnea directly. Your question is valid: if the stimulant medication helps this daytime sleepiness, why would you have to use the CPAP equipment? The most important thing to remember is that this stimulant medication does not prevent sleep apnea and the associated lowering of the blood oxygen saturation. Therefore, if you stop using the CPAP therapy, sleep apnea–related symptoms will come back; you will have repeated episodes when you will stop breathing during sleep and your blood oxygen saturation will be reduced below the normal levels, contributing to undesirable short- and long-term consequences.

56. Do I need retitration and retesting? If so, when and how would I know?

You should have a repeat overnight sleep study to find out if you have persistent sleep apnea, and if you do, you may need retitration to assess the pressure setting. In Question 54, it was mentioned that a certain percentage of asymptomatic patients have persistent sleep apnea, and the only way to uncover this is by doing an overnight sleep study. You should also be retested if you have had upper airway surgery or have been using oral appliances. Sleep apnea is a chronic illness; therefore it is important to retest to make sure the treatment is effective in order to prevent long-term adverse consequences. If your symptoms reappear after a period of being symptom free, if there is a change in your weight (you have either gained a considerable amount of weight or lost weight), or if you develop some other medical or neurological condition that might adversely affect the upper airway muscles, then you must have a repeat overnight sleep study and, if necessary, retitration to adjust the pressure setting of your CPAP unit.

57. How do I know if I am better after surgery or oral appliance?

After upper airway surgery or oral appliance you should begin to feel better within a few weeks, and gradually, two to three months after sufficient recovery from the surgery and after getting used to the oral appliance, you should remain symptom free. It is important to have a repeat overnight sleep study about three to four months after upper airway surgery or after oral appliance to make certain you do not have persistent sleep apnea. The procedures may have corrected your snoring and you may be under a false assumption that your sleep apnea has been completely eliminated.

58. How do I take care of my CPAP equipment?

Your home care company personnel should have given you instructions about the equipment and how to take care of it. If you did not get these instructions, call the company. I will briefly discuss some of the steps you should take to handle your machine, the mask, and the tubing. You must clean the mask daily by using warm, mild, soapy water, then rinse it and dry it. The tubing should be similarly cleaned weekly. To clean the humidifier, follow the manufacturer's directions and use sterile distilled water in the humidifier. The humidifier should generally be cleaned daily with mild, soapy water without using any chemicals. The manufacturers generally tell you to use a mixture of water and white vinegar to clean and disinfect the humidifier once a week. The distilled water not used during the night must be discarded each morning. The filter that comes with the equipment should be cleaned with mild soapy water and allowed to dry. The home care company generally advises changing the mask every six months. If the humidifier shows deposits inside after using for several months, it should be replaced with a new one. The main CPAP unit generally lasts for five to six years.

59. Does sleep apnea occur in children, and does it have similar symptoms and consequences as in adults?

Pediatricians and family physicians are beginning to be aware of the presence of sleep apnea in children. Children present with slightly different symptoms than adults. Children may not always have excessive daytime sleepiness as in adults but often present with abnormal daytime behavior, fatigue, inattention, impairment of school performance with lowering of school grades, hyperactivity resembling attention deficit/hyperactivity disorder (ADHD), morning headache, bed wetting, excessive sweating during sleep at night, restless sleep, excessive movements during sleep, frequent crying at night, noisy breathing at night, morning headache, mouth breathing, and sometimes episodes of sleep walking and nightmares. The most common cause of sleep apnea in children is enlarged tonsils causing partial obstruction of the upper airway in the back of the throat, giving rise to snoring and sleep apnea. Beware of a snoring, hyperactive child or a snoring, somnolent child and strongly suspect sleep apnea. The patient should be evaluated by having an overnight sleep study. It is important to make an early diagnosis to prevent problems in physical and mental growth because most children (at least 80% or better) show symptomatic improvement and cure of sleep apnea after tonsillectomy. In some patients, symptoms of sleep apnea may persist, and in those cases, surgery in the back of the throat in the region of the soft palate may help. A small percentage of children with sleep apnea may need CPAP therapy. It is important to monitor children with CPAP therapy very frequently and reevaluate every six months for mask fit because of rapid facial growth. Treating children with CPAP is difficult, and as a parent you must be educated in order to train your child to keep the mask on. Similar to the case with adults, weight loss should be encouraged because obesity is also very common in children with sleep apnea.

In a small percentage of children with sleep apnea, CPAP therapy is needed.

60. I am a pregnant woman in the second trimester of my pregnancy. Do I have an increased risk of developing sleep apnea?

Snoring is common in pregnancy, and there have been studies showing an increased prevalence of sleep apnea, particularly in the third trimester of pregnancy. Adequate prospective studies have not been performed to know the exact prevalence, but a small percentage of pregnant women develop sleep apnea as well as snoring. If you have snoring, especially loud snoring, accompanied by witnessed apneas and daytime sleepiness and fatigue, you should suspect sleep apnea and have an overnight sleep study to confirm the diagnosis because there are reports of growth retardation in the unborn babies of untreated sleep apneic pregnant women. Sleep apnea also increases your chances of developing high blood pressure and other pregnancy complications. If the diagnosis is confirmed, CPAP therapy should be instituted to correct the breathing events and to prevent further adverse consequences. Studies have shown that the symptoms of preexisting sleep apnea tend to increase during pregnancy in addition to a certain percentage of patients developing the symptoms of sleep apnea for the first time during pregnancy, especially in the third trimester.

Appendix

Resources

You can obtain essential information about sleep apnea from a number of professional and lay organizations. A number of Web sites disseminate valuable information about sleep and sleep disorders directed specifically at the public. This information has been written by doctors. In addition, many books are devoted to sleep medicine. The sources listed here should point you in the right direction.

American Academy of Sleep Medicine (AASM)
1 Westbrook Corporate Center
Suite 920
Westchester, IL 60154
Phone: (708) 492-0903

The mission of the AASM is to promote sleep disorders medicine to members of the medical and paramedical professions as well as to the public. The organization is dedicated to supporting quality care for patients with sleep disorders, providing public and professional education on the issues, and encouraging and supporting research in sleep medicine. The AASM on its Web site also lists the accredited sleep centers along with board-certified sleep medicine specialists on the staff of those centers.

American Sleep Apnea Association (ASAA)
www.sleepapnea.org
6856 Eastern Avenue, NW
Suite 203
Washington, DC 20012
Phone: (202) 293-3650
The ASAA is devoted to helping patients with sleep apnea and
works with a variety of support groups in the United States.
The ASAA also lists Alert, Well, and Keeping Energetic
(AWAKE) support groups in different states.

National Center for Sleep Disorders Research (NCSDR)
2 Rockledge Center
Suite 7024
6701 Rockledge Drive, MSC7920
Bethesda, MD 20892-7920
Phone: (301) 435-0199
The NCSDR was established after a national commission on
sleep disorders research, which was mandated by Congress,
recommended in 1993 that a national center for research and
education in sleep and sleep disorders be established. This center is located within the National Heart, Lung, and Blood
Institute of the National Institutes of Health (NIH) in
Bethesda, Maryland. It supports research, education, and train-
ing in sleep and sleep disorders for all health care professionals.
The center also participates in public awareness and education
campaigns about sleep disorders. It works in collaboration with
several federal agencies, including the NIH, the former Alcohol, Drug Abuse, and Mental Health Administration, and the
Departments of Defense, Transportation, and Veterans Affairs.

National Sleep Foundation (NSF)
729 Fifteenth Street, NW, 4th Floor
Washington, DC 20005
Phone: (202) 347-3471
The NSF produces valuable brochures dealing with sleep and
sleep disorders, promotes public education (particularly about
driving, fatigue, and sleepiness as well as important sleep disorders), and periodically organizes Gallup polls dealing with sleep
and sleep difficulties.

World Association of Sleep Medicine (WASM)
www.wasmonline.org
WASM Administrative Secretary
Klinikstr. 16
Kassel D-34128
Germany
Fax: 49-561-6009-126
E-mail: WASMsecretary[at]gmx.de
The fundamental mission of the WASM is to advance sleep
  health worldwide. WASM will fulfill its mission by promoting
  and encouraging education, research, and patient care throughout the world. WASM strives to advance knowledge about
  sleep and its disorders amongst both healthcare workers and
  the general public. WASM provides a forum for discussion and
  consideration of issues of relevance to particular regions and
  cultures. WASM has an online newsletter and the first issue
  deals with "Sleep Medicine Worldwide."

American Academy of Dental Sleep Medicine (AADSM)
www.dentalsleepmed.org
One Westbrook Corporate Center Suite 920
Westchester, IL 60154
Phone: (708) 273-9366
Fax: (708) 492-0943
The mission of the AADSM is to promote the use and resource
  of oral appliances and oral surgeries for the treatment of sleep
  apnea.

List of CPAP Manufacturers

ResMed Corporation

Philips Respironics

Puritan Bennet

Fisher Paykel

There are some CPAP Internet stores.

Recommended Books

Berry RB, ed. Sleep medicine pearls. 2nd ed. Philadelphia: Henley and Belfus, 2003.

Chokroverty S. Clinical companion to sleep disorders medicine. Boston: Butterworth/Elsevier.

Chokroverty S. One hundred questions and answers about sleep disorders. 2nd ed. Boston: Jones and Bartlett.

Chokroverty S., ed. Sleep disorders medicine: basic science, technical considerations and clinical aspects. Philadelphia: Butterworth/Elsevier.

Kryger MH, Roth T, Dement WC, eds. Principles and practice of sleep medicine. Philadelphia: Elsevier/Saunders.

Lee-Chiung TL, ed. Sleep: a comprehensive handbook. Hoboken, NJ: Wiley.

Silber MH, Krah LE, Morgenthaler TI, eds. Sleep medicine in clinical practice. Boca Raton, FL: Taylor and Francis.

Glossary

Acetylcholine: The main chemical agent causing activation of REM sleep.

Acid regurgitation: Condition in which acid from the stomach flows back into the esophagus.

Adenoids: Lymphoid tissues in the throat behind the nasal passage.

Adherence: Willingness to continue with long-term therapy.

Amyotrophic lateral sclerosis (ALS): *See Lou Gehrig's Disease*

Autonomic nervous system: The part of the nervous system controlling vital functions of the body such as circulation, respiration, and hormone secretion.

Bariatric surgery: Procedure performed to assist obese patients in achieving weight loss.

Bi-level therapy: A CPAP device that can be adjusted so that it delivers higher-pressure air during inhalation and lower-pressure air during expiration.

Brain stem: Deeper part in the base of the brain which connects the main brain hemisphere with the spinal cord.

Central sleep apnea (CSA): Abnormal breathing during sleep, wherein the airflow stops at the nose and mouth and the breathing effort by the diaphragm (the main muscle of breathing) and other muscles of aspiration stops.

Confusional arousals: Episodes that may occur during deep dreamless sleep involving complex behaviors without conscious awareness.

Continuous positive airway pressure (CPAP): Remedial therapy involving a small portable machine used to deliver air through the nose to the back of the throat.

CPAP device: A CPAP device includes a mask, head straps, tubes, and a fan. It reduces snoring and prevents apnea disturbances.

CPAP mask: An interface with head straps and a valve to adjust the pressure of the air delivered through the nose into the back of the throat.

CPAP titration: A gradual adjusting of the flow of air until the desired effect is achieved.

Diaphragm: The main muscle of breathing, located at the junction of the chest and abdomen.

Electroencephalogram (EEG): A recording of the electrical activities of the brain.

Electromyogram (EMG): A recording of the electrical activities of the muscles.

Electro-oculogram (EOG): A recording of the movements of the eye.

Emphysema: Excessive stretching of the lungs.

Epworth Sleepiness Scale: A tool used during diagnostic processes to assess subjective evidence of sleepiness.

Expiration: Exhaling air during breathing.

Flow generator: The part of CPAP therapy that delivers room air at a positive pressure.

Heart failure: The inability of the heart to pump blood adequately to different body regions.

Hemoglobin: Blood pigment, the color of which indicates blood oxygen saturation.

Homeostasis: Maintenance of internal equilibrium which ensures that a period of wakefulness is followed by a sleep debt and a propensity to sleep.

Humidifier: A device that adds humidity to breathed air to prevent drying of nasal passages.

Hypersomnia: Recurrent episodes of excessive daytime sleepiness or prolonged nighttime sleep.

Hypopnea: Reduction of breathing volume to below the normal level.

Increment: To increase or add, as observed in certain chemicals during sleep deprivation.

Lou Gehrig's disease: Amyotrophic lateral sclerosis (ALS). A serious condition characterized by progressive death of nerve cells controlling muscles of the body.

Microsleep: Transient periods of NREM stage 1 sleep occuring during sleep deprivation experiments.

Micturition: Function of urination, increased frequency of which interferes with sleep.

Mixed apnea: Abnormal breathing during sleep, characterized by an initial period of central apnea, followed by a period of obstructive apnea.

Multiple daytime sleep study: A very important test to assess the severity of daytime sleepiness.

Multiple sleep latency (MSLT): A scoring system used to determine objective evidence of sleepiness.

Narcolepsy: A sleep disorder characterized by excessive daytime sleepiness.

Nightmare: Vivid and frightening dreams, also known as dream anxiety attack.

Non-rapid eye movement (NREM) sleep: A multi-stage phase of the progression from wakefulness into deep sleep.

Obstructive sleep apnea (OSA): Abnormal breathing during sleep, wherein the passage of inhaled air becomes obstructed in the region of the upper airway.

Parkinson Disease (PD): A degenerative disorder of the central nervous system that often impairs the sufferer's motor skills and speech.

Partial arousal disorder: A condition in which the body is apparently active, but the brain is confused and only partially awakened.

Pillar procedure: Surgery on the palate in which polyester rods are implanted into the soft palate.

Pituitary gland: The organ responsible for secretion of several important hormones.

Poliomyelitis: The inflammation of the spinal cord, often called Infantile Paralysis.

Polysomnographic study: An overnight laboratory test used to diagnose primary sleep problems.

Post-polio syndrome: Weakness of arm or leg formerly affected by poliomyelitis, accompanied by paralysis of muscles, including those of the previously unaffected extremities, and often breathing difficulties.

Predormitum: A state of diminished perception and control through which a person passes in progressing from wakefulness into the sleep state.

Rapid eye movement (REM) sleep: The stage of sleep during which dreaming occurs.

Retina: The layer of nerve cells at the back of the eye responsible for transmitting visual images to the back of the brain.

Serotonin: One of the chemicals responsible for inactivation of REM sleep.

Sleep apnea: A very serious sleep disturbing condition in which a sleeper stops breathing for at least 10 seconds several times during the night, resulting in interruptions of the sleep cycle.

Sleep deprivation: A condition of sleeplessness resulting in sleep debt and other adverse consequences.

Sleep latency: Defined as the time elapsed between lights off and the first onset of any stage of sleep as determined by the changes in brain wave activity.

Sleep onset insomnia: A sleep disorder in which the patient is unable to fall asleep for long periods, resulting in insufficient rest and daytime tiredness.

Sleep spindles: Brain rhythms of 14 to 16 cycles per second that are seen in surface recordings taken from the front and center of the head during NREM sleep.

Snoring: Noisy sound generated by an obstruction to the free flow of air through the passages at the back of the mouth and nose caused by vibration of the uvula and soft palate during sleep, contributing to reduction of sleep quality.

Soft palate: Soft, muscular tissue in the back of the roof of the mouth.

Suprachiasmatic nuclei: A cluster of nerve cells within which the human internal clock is thought to reside.

Temporomandibular joint: The jaw joint.

Titration: The adjustment made to the CPAP flow generator to deliver optimal pressure level to eliminate sleep disordered breathing events.

Tolerance: Reduction in effect of a drug and need for higher doses to produce adequate effect.

Tonsils: Areas of lymphoid tissue on either side of the throat.

Transient insomnia: Also known as short-term or acute insomnia, resulting from an identifiable stressful situation.

Uvula: The small piece of soft pear-shaped structure that can be seen dangling down from the soft palate over the back of the tongue.

Video-polysomnographic study: Continuous video monitoring during a sleep study which measures physiological characteristics, correlating these with the behavior of the individual.

Zeitgebers: External time-givers removed during laboratory time-isolation experiments.

Index